Make Chronic Disease

Your Guide to Living Pain Free Through Functional Medicine

Remember to Call:
Trish Murray, DO
Empowering People to Live a Pain Free Life
(603) 447-3112
Discoverhealthfmc.com
trishmurraydo@gmail.com

Mary —
To Your Health!

Trish Murray DO

Make a D.E.N.T.™ in Chronic Disease

Your Guide to Living Pain Free Through Functional Medicine

Trish Murray, DO

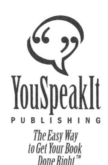

YouSpeakIt
PUBLISHING
The Easy Way
to Get Your Book
Done Right™

www.YouSpeakItPublishing.com

*Dedicated to you who are dealing with
chronic health conditions, searching for answers,
and willing to make choices that can empower you
to optimize and restore your health.*

Contents

Acknowledgments

Many people have been a part of my life journey and have given me insight:

My parents; my brothers and my sister; my partner, Elaine; my children, Ben and Shea; my patients; my friends; my colleagues; and all my staff.

Every relationship, every interaction has been a piece of my learning puzzle. Thank you!

Introduction

You have the power to change your life and optimize your own health. My mission is to empower you with education, community, and support to bring you to your greatest state of well-being.

Our traditional medical system has been based on how to treat acute disease, infections, injuries, and physical traumas. If you have a gall bladder attack, the medical model's approach is to surgically remove it; if you've broken a bone, doctors can set the bone to help you heal. Today's medical model is successful at interventions for acute conditions.

The healthcare problem of our time, however, is chronic disease. Many people are living day in and day out with chronic conditions. In my local area, 59 percent of people over fifty-five years old have three or more chronic diseases that they take medication for daily. This is not a unique statistic, and the medical model treatment mentality is to prescribe a pill for every ill.

The doctor does a physical exam, checks labs, and when you meet with them for the results of your lab work, they tell you everything is normal and everything is fine.

You hear this news in awe, and say, "Okay, but I still don't feel well."

So at this point, the doctor does what they are trained to do and prescribes medications to alleviate or mask your different symptoms, but this doesn't work.

The good news is that another form of medicine is growing more every day: *functional medicine*. Functional medicine focuses on exactly how your body works and how the different systems interrelate. It's also called *root cause* medicine. This book will help you look for the root causes of the imbalances or the dysfunctions within the systems of your body.

The most common root causes of chronic disease are inflammation or imbalance in the immune system. If your immune system is out of balance, and the dysfunction has continued for too long, then your immune system is going to start turning against you, and you may develop what's called an *autoimmune disease*.

Now, understanding the root cause of how your body functions takes a great deal of education. In addition to teaching you about your immune system, this book explores how the acute disease model of the traditional medical system—of just giving you another pill, or taking out one of your organs with surgery—does not get at the dysfunction that's causing the problem. This book helps you understand that you have the power to bring your immune system back into balance and decrease inflammation. You can heal your chronic conditions with the choices you make in life.

I have seen people improve their chronic diseases and heal themselves with the knowledge we share in my practice. For several years, we have been teaching a curriculum I developed, named D.E.N.T.™.

D.E.N.T.™ is an acronym for:

- Diet and Detox
- Exercise
- Nutrition
- Treatment

When you come to us for healthcare, we begin by asking you to fill out a *medical symptoms questionnaire*. That medical symptoms questionnaire addresses symptoms throughout all the different systems of your body. The questionnaire helps us pinpoint which systems are problematic. You score yourself based on the symptoms you experience. Optimal health is represented by a score less than thirty. If you score more than thirty, that means you have some level of dysfunction in your systems. Some of the people I have worked with started with a score of *more than a hundred*.

After you learn the concepts I share in this book and come to understand how diet, exercise, and nutrition are foundational to your health, you can reduce your score to less than thirty, improve your health, and live longer, stronger, and healthier. It is not through taking another pill. It is through making certain changes and choices about how you're living your life and the environment in which you live.

I want you to realize that your life choices strengthen or weaken your immune system:

- What foods do you eat?
- How do you perceive stress, and how do you manage it?
- Do you get enough rest?
- Do you include movement in every day?
- What chemicals do you clean your home with and put on your body?

Every choice makes a difference.

If there is imbalance in your immune system, inflammation and toxicity will develop and set the stage for the development and progression of most chronic dis-eases. But it doesn't have to be this way.

When you finish this book, you will understand the different environmental choices that you can make, you will be empowered, and you will be able to make changes in your life to feel better and to bring balance into your world.

CHAPTER ONE

Root Causes—Immune Imbalances and Inflammation

In the practice of tolerance, one's enemy is the best teacher.
~ His Holiness the 14th Dalai Lama

HOW THE IMMUNE SYSTEM WORKS

The immune system is an extremely complex system to understand, so I'm going to break it down into parts. Your immune system is your defense system. It's your military: your navy, your air force, your marines, your police. Its responsibility is to keep you safe in your world.

Once any foreign substance enters your body, your immune system goes into action to protect you by initiating your *innate immune system*. It sends in ground forces as your first line of defense against any invader or threat. The cells of your innate immune system initiate battle against any infection, but they also train your adaptive immune system to send in reinforcements during the battle against any invader. So, your immune system has multiple levels of defense.

Stranger Danger

We live in a dangerous world in which we're exposed to many health risks:

- Chemicals
- Bacteria
- Viruses
- Molds
- Toxins
- Injuries
- Stress

You can think of these risks as threats to the optimal health of your body, like invaders or strangers. In our external world, we talk about *stranger danger* as having an awareness of potential threats from people we don't know. We teach our children not to talk to strangers, and we keep alert in situations that seem to be risky if someone uninvited or unrecognized approaches.

If there is a threat to your internal environment—for example, through a wound or cut in your skin— your innate immune system sends in ground forces in response to this immediate stranger danger. This initial response to any invader comes from our innate immune system and typically involves inflammation.

Everyone is familiar with inflammation. Whenever you cut your finger or sprain your ankle, for example, the area of the injury hurts and becomes swollen, red, and warm. The body part also may not function normally. These are the typical external signs we see and feel when inflammation is present.

But, when the injury or threat is internal, it's a different experience. You can't see the inflammation because it lives below the surface of your skin. Internal inflammation of your nervous system, digestive system, or another of your organs can occur below the surface of your skin like an iceberg. You may have some signs or symptoms that you are aware of *above the surface,* but a much larger mass or level of inflammation lives below the surface so you are not aware of its true size.

The ground forces of your innate immune system go into action whenever any dangerous bug, trauma, or injury occurs. Its first job is to engage any foreign invader and destroy it.

How exactly do they accomplish this?

There are different ways that the innate immune cells can try to destroy the stranger danger. All innate immune cells contain chemicals that can be used as weapons when they are in danger.

Another defense your ground forces employ is *phagocytosis,* in which an innate immune cell—a *phagocyte,* from *phag,* meaning "eat" and *cyte,* meaning "cell"—engulfs a bacterium, virus, or chemical, and devours it.

If your ground forces of your innate immune system cannot eliminate any invader completely, then they have a third method of protection. They can place signals on their membranes that can train reinforcements—*adaptive* immune cells—how to identify the enemy.

These signals communicate to the *adaptive immune system: We have a stranger in the house and we need more help!*

Here Come the Reinforcements

Once the innate immune cells attack the stranger danger and engage it in battle, they also place chemical receptors on their own membranes that they then present to your naive adaptive immune cells. This information activates your adaptive immune system and delivers crucial information about the enemy.

The naive adaptive cells are trained to look for these signals and then attack. The adaptive immune system cells are your reinforcements. They come in as a second form of attack. However, this takes time. Your innate immune system reacts for the first ninety hours, but the adaptive immune system takes four to five days to come into play. Once it's in place, it will have long-term memories of what to attack and what to kill. The virus you have today takes seven to ten days to get rid of. Your innate immune system comes into play immediately, and then your adaptive immune system takes four to five days to be trained and activated. Then, the two systems work in full force to eradicate and neutralize any invader or toxin.

The cells of the adaptive immune system, while they are being activated by the signals from the innate immune system cells, can be trained into one of two different pathways or branches of your military. In the same way that a soldier can enlist in the navy or the air force, an adaptive immune cell can be enlisted into one of two branches of the active adaptive immune system. It could go down a Th1 pathway. This Th1 branch of your adaptive immune system activates T-cell mediated activation of macrophages and neutrophils, whereas the Th2 pathway activates a B-cell mediated activation of mast cells, eosinophils, and basophils.

If your adaptive immune system becomes hypersensitive and overreactive, it can initiate an autoimmune reaction against *self*—your own tissues. If hypersensitivity and dysfunction happen to your Th1 adaptive immune cells, then particular autoimmune disease processes develop, such as rheumatoid arthritis, multiple sclerosis, Crohn's disease, and thyroid-related disease. If the Th2 branch becomes dysfunctional, then more allergy-related diseases develop, such as asthma, eczema, and psoriasis.

We Must Have Tolerance

This complex system, which consists of an innate immune system and an adaptive, trained immune system with long-term memory, must also have tolerance. For example, imagine you are sitting on your front porch, and all of a sudden you hear some weird noise. You look down the street, and you see a group of strange people walking down the sidewalk of your neighborhood.

You think: *What the heck are they doing?*

You notice that the hairs on the back of your neck go up, and you're quite alarmed.

Then, your son or daughter walks out to the porch and says, "Hey Charlie, John, Susie! How are you doing?" and they wave to this group of people.

Now, you realize these strangers are your child's friends. The hairs on the back of your neck go down, you're no longer nervous, and you're no longer scared. You now have tolerance.

Well, your immune system does this constantly. If your innate immune cells have seen a foreign substance before, and it's never caused danger, then they let each other know to tolerate that substance's presence.

On the other hand, let's say you're sitting on the porch and the same situation occurs. A group of people is walking toward you, down the sidewalk of your neighborhood, making strange noises, and acting differently. You stand up to get a better look and you're nervous. The hair goes up on your neck, and all of a sudden, your daughter, son, or spouse comes out, and they see this group of people. They don't know the group, either.

They say, "What the heck is going on? Who is that?"

Now you're both scared. You're both nervous. You both start reacting to this stranger danger, and you're watching. You start moving to get a better look at the strangers and start contemplating your next move to stay safe and protect yourself and your family.

You may call the police.

You may go out and possibly question these people yourself.

In this situation, tolerance does not exist. You're more concerned. You want to know why these people are in your neighborhood, and if they are dangerous, then you're going to act.

In the end, you must be able to discern whether something is true stranger danger or not. Your immune system is constantly trying to figure this out before it reacts.

IMMUNE SYSTEM IMBALANCES CAN HIDE BELOW THE SURFACE

So many of us go through our daily life and don't feel well.

Do you feel like you are as productive as you could be?

Do you feel like your brain is working with optimal abilities?

If your answer to the above questions isn't yes, it could be that there are imbalances in your body and that underlying inflammation is causing these problems. I'd like to help you understand why this is so and what indicators to look for to determine if your immune system may be out of balance.

"But All My Labs Are Normal"

So many of my patients have come to me with the same story. They had consulted their primary care practitioner and complained that they weren't feeling well. Their symptoms included fatigue, no weight loss — regardless of what they did or ate — chronic joint pain, headaches, insomnia, and mood swings. The primary care provider did basic blood work and in the follow-up meeting, their provider reported that labs were completely normal.

Their primary care doctor said: *I have great news for you: Your labs are normal! You're healthy!*

But these people still didn't feel well.

One of my patients, whom I'll call Jackie, came to me with complaints of fatigue and anxiety. Essentially, she felt wired and tired all the time. One year before, she had gone to her primary care provider (PCP) with the complaint of feeling tired. The blood work that was done was all in the normal ranges. Particularly, all her thyroid-related numbers were normal. But in order to try to help, her PCP prescribed a low dose of thyroid medication to see if it would help her fatigue. Since taking the prescription medication, the patient continued to feel tired but additionally felt wired and anxious.

This case is a good example of the fact that prescription medications are essentially the only tool that the traditional medical model uses to treat symptoms. I was originally trained in this model and practiced as a PCP in internal medicine. Many times, I felt like all I was doing was pushing pills and dealing with side effects to those pills. As a result, I went searching for other answers and found functional medicine, which has taught me to go back to my training in biochemical and physiologic pathways to identify the root cause of each person's systemic dysfunctions.

The bottom line is normal labs don't mean that everything is normal for every patient. There could be underlying inflammation. There could be an underlying autoimmune imbalance. Multiple systems in the body can be off without tipping the lab values that most traditional healthcare practitioners measure.

Jackie ended up going through my D.E.N.T.™ Program and as a result, learned that she was sensitive to gluten and dairy. Once she removed these from her diet, her energy improved, and she no longer felt wired all the time. This is the perfect example of how factors in our daily environment can be root causes of our systemic imbalance.

Complex Symptoms Are Clues to Chronic Immune Imbalances

We all have symptoms from time to time. But when you have a collection of related symptoms, they are signs or clues that you have immune imbalances.

Typical symptoms of immune imbalances include:

- Chronic pain
- Fatigue
- Hair thinning or loss
- Depression
- Anxiety
- Mood swings
- Insomnia
- Cold hands and feet
- Inexplicable weight gain
- Night sweats

The list of symptoms for immune system dysfunction can be extremely complex.

The last fifty years of traditional, standard medical care has developed so that most practitioners faced with a list of complex symptoms will prescribe you a pill for every ill. With multiple prescriptions, the side effects of all those pills are not going to cause improved health; instead, they are likely to cause more symptoms, more complexity, more problems, and more pain.

If you are experiencing numerous symptoms, they are your clues that below the surface, there is immune imbalance, and there is an iceberg that needs to be melted.

Anxiety and Depression Are Really Inflamed Brains

The systems of your body are extremely complicated, and you have multiple systems that make you who you are, including:

- Nervous system
- Gastrointestinal system
- Pulmonary system
- Respiratory system
- Immune system

They must all work in unison and in balance. If your immune system is constantly out of balance and constantly fighting against each thing that it sees as if it is a stranger danger, then you are going to have inflammation in your body. But, as mentioned before, you're not going to see this on the surface like a cut or a skin wound. Instead, this inflammation is growing and spreading below the surface, like an iceberg.

One of the primary systems affected by inflammation is your nervous system — which includes your brain. Your brain is an organ like any other organ, and it becomes inflamed when the immune system is out of balance. Anxiety, depression, and cognitive decline are now understood to be directly related to underlying inflammation, autoimmunity, and immune imbalances in the body.

The field of psychiatry, which over the last fifty years has relied predominantly on medications, is starting to acknowledge the connection between emotional wellness, brain health, and the physical body. The connection between leaky gut, inflammation, toxicity, and one's brain function is supported more and more by research.

THE CONSEQUENCES OF DISRUPTING OUR PROTECTIVE BARRIERS

For the last fifty or more years, we've been told that we get our genes from our mother and father, and that our genes are our destiny. Your doctor probably begins assessing your health by taking your family history and emphasizing that you are destined to develop the diseases of your parents. But scientific research of the last twenty years has shown that your genetic makeup is not necessarily your destiny.

Your Genes Are Not Your Destiny

Auto means "self," and when your imbalanced immune system attacks *self*, that means it's attacking *you* — your healthy cells as well as any stranger danger. Autoimmune diseases can attack your nervous system, resulting in anxiety, depression, or cognitive decline;

or your endocrine system, as with thyroid gland issues like Hashimoto's disease.

There are three factors present in the development of an autoimmune disease:

1. Genetic susceptibility
2. Environmental triggers
3. Barrier dysfunction

Your genes are not the only, nor the most important, aspect of this problem.

There is a concept called *epigenetics*. The prefix *epi-* means on, upon, or above, so epigenetics means the science *above* the genes. This means that a person's daily environment, such as the foods they eat, whether they move and exercise, and their stress level, affects their genetics. Recent research suggests that epigenetics is the most important aspect of your health.

There have been studies on identical twins that generally confirm that genes aren't everything.[1] Let's say there are two identical twins, Johnny and Bobby. Both boys grow up in a supportive environment, but when they become adults, they make different lifestyle choices. Bobby's relationships are strong. He doesn't

---

1   Bell, J. and T. Spector. "A Twin Approach to Unraveling Epigenetics." *Trends in Genetics.* 2011 Mar; 27(3): 116–125. DOI: 10.106/j.tig.2010.005

drink alcohol, he doesn't use drugs, and he eats very healthy foods. His brother, Johnny, makes opposite choices. If we were to follow these two identical twins through their lives, we would find their health would be very different. They would have different illnesses and respond differently to disease, injury, or trauma. Observations such as these have been noted as proof of the concept of epigenetics and the idea that our environment is much more powerful in our overall health than our genetics.

In a 2013 article in *The Guardian,* author Robin McKie includes this further explanation from Professor Tim Spector, head of twin research at King's College in London:

> Essentially, epigenetics is the mechanism by which environmental changes alter the behaviour of our genes. . . . This involves a process known as methylation, which occurs when a chemical known as methyl, which floats around the inside of our cells, attaches itself to our DNA. When it does so, it can inhibit or turn down the activity of a gene and block it from making a particular version of a protein in our bodies.

McKie goes on to say that, "Crucially, all sorts of life events can affect DNA methylation levels in our bodies:

diet, illnesses, aging, chemicals in the environment, smoking, drugs, and medicines."[2]

The environmental factors that can epigenetically affect your genes include:

- The foods you eat
- The cosmetics you put on your skin
- The medications you take
- The alcohol you drink
- The choices you make every day
- The stress you experience and how you deal with it
- The relationships you're in and how they feed you or drain you

As we've discussed before, many of these elements are within your control, and you can choose deliberately to take a path toward better health.

The third factor concerns healthy *barriers*, the structures that keep the outside world out and your inside world in. They make up your fort. Your skin, for example, is an obvious barrier that protects you from the outside world. We are all aware of how our skin is meant to protect us from the outside world whenever we get a

---

2   McKie, Robin. "Why Do Identical Twins End Up Having Such Different Lives?" *The Guardian*. June 1, 2013. theguardian. com/science/2013/jun/02/twins-identical-genes-different-health-study

cut. The first thing we notice is that we start bleeding and we need to stop this by applying a bandage and some pressure, but the second most important thing we do is to clean the wound and apply some antiseptic or antibiotic because we know that our skin barrier has been damaged and dangerous bugs or infection-causing chemicals now have the opportunity to enter our body.

Another barrier is the wall of your digestive tract. You may have heard about *leaky gut syndrome,* but you may not know what it means. The gastrointestinal system is a hose that runs from your mouth to your stomach, then on to your small intestines. Your small intestines then become the colon, then the rectum, and end with the anus.

The wall of this hose is a barrier. When you take food into your mouth, that's taking something from the outside world and putting it inside. The food during digestion gets broken down into different components, some of which we absorb through the wall of our intestines as nutrients and others that are waste products or toxins that are not meant to absorb through the wall or barrier of our intestines.

For example, through the cells of our intestinal wall, we are meant to absorb vitamins, minerals, proteins, fats, and carbohydrates at their most elemental form;

but, we are not supposed to absorb fiber or bacteria or chemicals.

The lining of your digestive tract, the inside wall of this hose, is a layer with the thickness equivalent to only one cell. That one-cell layer is very susceptible to injury if you don't feed it well and keep it strong. The cells that make up the thin layer have very tight junctions between them when you are healthy. But they can be damaged, creating gaps between those cells. As you can imagine, these gaps allow substances to leak through the wall, and that is what causes a leaky gut.

Another important barrier in our bodies is the *blood-brain barrier*. Over a century ago, it was discovered that blue dye injected into the bloodstream would cause the tissues of the whole body — except the brain and spinal column — to turn blue. It was then realized that there are high-density cells that line the capillaries, or smallest blood vessels, feeding the brain. These cells restrict passage of substances from the bloodstream much more than the cells in the capillaries elsewhere in the body and act as a barrier to protect the brain from foreign substances.[3]

---

3   Obermeier, B., R. Daneman, and R. M. Ransohoff. "Development, Maintenance and Disruption of the Blood-Brain Barrier." *Nature Medicine*. 19(12), 1584–1596. 2013. DOI: 10.1038/nm.3407

Keep the Fort Strong

Right behind the wall of the fort is your military, your ground forces, and your army. As we have said, your immune system is your military, so it makes sense that the majority of your immune system, 80 percent, sits right behind your gut wall. If you have a leaky gut, damaging bacteria and harmful chemicals can travel through that leaky gut. If this is the case, your immune system will be constantly reacting to different invaders and become hypersensitive and overreactive. This barrier dysfunction and immune system hypersensitivity typically is the root cause of inflammation and autoimmunity.

Your Day-to-Day Choices Are More Powerful Than You Realize

The choices you make every day create your environment. You make and create the environment you live in, and those choices bring information to your immune system, your gut, and to your entire body. For example, food is a form of information. Food that is nutritious and healthy will give you good information. Food that is not healthy will give your body and your immune system bad information.

Jackie, the patient I mentioned earlier, came to me for help with figuring out thyroid medicine, anxiety, and feeling wired all the time. For a treatment plan, we started with food; we always start with food. You put food in your mouth and into your system, and it is your fuel, more than any other substance.

We guided Jackie through a three-week detox. Prior to doing the detox, she noted many symptoms throughout her body on the medical symptoms questionnaire. She scored more than 100 points — about 130 — which is extremely high. A person in optimal health typically scores less than thirty total points on the medical symptoms questionnaire. On the three-week detox, Jackie restricted certain foods that can be highly inflammatory and common triggers in the environment. She cleaned up her diet in a very specific way.

After simply making deliberate choices about food daily, her medical symptoms questionnaire score went down to twenty-four. Her anxiety improved, she was sleeping through the night, and she felt stronger and more energetic.

While food is only one facet of your health, it's a huge piece of the overall picture. Other pieces can be looked at, evaluated, and cleaned up as well.

The big idea here is that every day you make choices, and those choices impact your well-being:

- What cosmetics do you use?
- Are your house cleaners and detergents nontoxic?
- Do you eat nourishing foods?
- Do you get enough rest?
- Is movement a part of each day?
- Do you use recreational drugs or alcohol?
- What is your stress level and how do you relieve it?

If you learn how to clean up your lifestyle and environment and dedicate yourself to that practice, then you will significantly improve your health, balance your immune system, and melt that iceberg.

I first came to see Trish Murray, DO, because I needed help with metabolic syndrome. I have high blood pressure, high cholesterol, and diabetes. It seemed every time I went to my primary care doctor that I would need to add another prescription, and my numbers were getting worse and worse, and I was tired of taking more pills. I wanted to take a different approach. And I am more than amazed at the results that I have had!

I joined the group that Dr. Murray started and within three days, I felt like a new person. At the end of four months, I feel as though I am totally transformed and have my life and my health back!

I think that Functional Medicine looks at you in a different way. I think it looks at the whole person. I think it believes in education and teaching you why you feel the way you do and why you need to make changes in your life to make yourself feel better. I can't say enough good things about the journey that I have been on with the support of everybody on the staff at Discover Health Functional Medicine Center.

~ Jeanne Primeau

CHAPTER TWO

The Environment You Create Supports Balance or Imbalance

We make the world we live in
and shape our own environment.
~ Orison Swett Marden

YOU ARE MORE IN CONTROL OF YOUR HEALTH THAN YOU THINK

In the first chapter, we talked about the complexity of the immune system. There are three things that need to happen to develop an autoimmune disease process, hypersensitivity, or imbalance in the immune system:

- Genetic susceptibility
- Environmental triggers
- Barrier dysfunction

In this chapter, I focus on the *modifiable factors* in your life: the elements you control in your environment that strengthen your forces, empower you, heal you, and heal your barriers or can weaken you, create illness, and cause dis-ease.

Environmental Triggers

There are so many different *triggers,* or environmental factors, that can either empower and strengthen your life, health, and fort, or can throw you off balance and cause your immune system to constantly be hyperactive and hypervigilant:

1. **Food.** We put food in our mouths multiple times a day. Any food could be an allergen, which you might notice immediately. Allergic *reactions* to foods, like hives, itchy eyes, difficulty breathing, or diarrhea, happen immediately. Many people do not understand that a *sensitivity* to a food might not appear for hours to days after eating a particular food. Some symptoms of food sensitivities include brain fog and headache, gas, abdominal discomfort, joint pain, acne breakouts, and irritability.

2. **Toxins.** We are all exposed to many toxins simply by living in our present world. Some of these toxins you have choice about and some you don't. Exhaust from traffic, cleansers in

public buildings, and contaminated municipal water are examples of the factors that are out of your control. Alcohol intake, soaps, cleaning products, and the cosmetics you use are examples of products that are within your control and choice.

3. **Infections.** You can be exposed to acute infections that can become chronic. Viruses spread through public spaces such as grocery stores, mass transit, and gyms are not difficult to pick up if your immune system is not strong. Lyme disease, Epstein-Barr virus, and molds are examples of infections that can become chronic and hide from your immune system.

4. **Stress** is another environmental trigger. Trauma, such as physical injury or sudden loss, can cause stress. Stress can also be caused by an acute environmental trigger, such as a natural disaster. Most of us are exposed to daily chronic stress due to our jobs, financial situation, or relationships — which is a particularly dangerous form of stress because it is constant and never-ending. Healthy stress is meant to occur and challenge us to fight, flee, or excel in something, but then to resolve so we can relax. Chronic, never-ending stress is extremely unhealthy.

5. **Allergens** other than food, such as pollen, mold, dust, and cigarette smoke, can trigger reactions.

6. **Relationships.** Does your primary relationship support you or drain you? Some relationships feel like they take more energy than they give. If you need to guard yourself when you're around someone, that can be exhausting work that depletes and compromises your immune system.

7. **Drugs.** If you choose to imbibe alcohol, take recreational drugs, or smoke cigarettes, you already know these are toxins of choice. Prescription medications also can be beneficial or detrimental. If a you are on multiple daily medications, they all may have interactions and must be metabolized and detoxified by your body.

Day-to-Day Choices

When you consider the environmental triggers listed above, I hope you realize that you can provide all the systems of your body, especially the immune system, with either bad information, or with good, healthy, strengthening information.

You must keep your *military* — your immune function — strong. If you don't, then your fort and your soldiers will break down. Your day-to-day choices—all the environmental triggers and the choices you make about each one of them—are either going to empower you or sicken you.

Your Microbiome and Your Health

We live in a symbiotic relationship with bacteria or bugs.

Bacteria live with you throughout your body:

- On your skin
- In your sinuses
- In your eyes
- In your gut

Bacteria live all over and through you, and they must be there in order for your body to be healthy. These bugs make up your microbiome, and it is very important to have this community of beneficial, health-promoting bacteria. You see, your microbiome is like a neighborhood. You want a good gang running the neighborhood, a gang that's going to help you be healthy. And your diet, stress, toxins, and so on are all extremely important in determining whether a health-promoting gang of bacteria or a disease-promoting gang of bacteria are running the neighborhood.

You want to keep the bad gangs out of town if you can. But the whole concept of using antibiotics *everywhere* in the industrialized world, like in soap, shampoo, and hand wipes, causes autoimmune disease. Third-world countries do not have even close to the rate of autoimmune disease that the industrialized population does in the world.

Yes, bacteria can cause illness and infection, but only certain bad bacteria. The beneficial ones actually promote good health, and we need them because without them, we would be dead.

So, ask yourself: *Do my lifestyle choices promote the right bacteria to be living in my microbiome and running the neighborhood, or the wrong bacteria to be determining my health and running the neighborhood?*

Think about it: If you make choices every day to feed your body and your microbiome what it needs to be strong and healthy, then you will be strong and healthy. If you make choices that weaken or sicken your microbiome and your own systems, then you will also experience weakness and illness.

Little Changes Make a Big Difference

Melora is forty-three years old, and when she first came to me, she shared with me, "My immune system has never functioned like other people's."

She suffered with allergies and hives, migraine headaches, and constipation since she was a small child. As an adult, she suffers with fatigue due to insomnia; she never sleeps through the night. She has hypothyroidism and recently developed heart palpitations and an abnormal heart rhythm, which has caused her to develop shortness of breath when she exercises. On her original medical symptoms questionnaire, our intake form described in the first chapter, she scored a sixty-three at first. Optimal health is to score less than thirty.

She started our D.E.N.T.™ Program. D.E.N.T.™ is an acronym that stands for:

- Diet and detox
- Exercise
- Nutrition
- Treatment

When we begin the D.E.N.T.™ Program with a patient, we initially recommend a diet following what I call the *Rainbow Concept*:

1. Eat real food of all the colors of the rainbow: red, yellow, orange, green, blue, and purple.

2. Decrease grains to only one or two servings per day.

3. Increase healthy fats: olive oil, coconut oil or coconut milk, avocado, nuts.

4. Limit sweets and desserts to one per week (yes, that *does* read one per week!).

Melora already followed a pretty healthy diet when she joined my program, so did not experience much difference in her health status with the rainbow concepts alone. But the other part of the "D" in our D.E.N.T.™ curriculum, however, is for detox, which is essentially a three-week elimination diet. During this time, all the foods that are the most typical triggers for food allergies or sensitivities are eliminated from the diet.

These foods include items such as:

- Gluten
- Dairy
- Soy
- Sugar
- Peanuts
- Night shade vegetables (tomatoes, peppers, eggplant, and potatoes)
- Alcohol

Six weeks into the D.E.N.T.™ Program, Melora had a number of reasons why she wasn't ready to do the elimination yet. She had a birthday party coming up, a holiday, and a wedding.

I said to her, "You know, you've been sick for a really long time. Don't you think it's time to get into this detox?"

She finally initiated her detox and eight weeks later, she reported:

- She no longer has any hives.

- She is one month off all allergy medications.

- Her medical symptoms questionnaire has dropped to a twenty-nine, which is now at a level of optimal health.

- Her energy is better.

- She is sleeping better.

- She seems extremely empowered and hopeful.

Even more awesome, Melora has a seven-year-old daughter. Actually, she has three daughters, but her seven-year-old daughter was extremely sick, not gaining weight, and had abdominal problems. She had her daughter and her whole family do the detox together and as a result, her daughter no longer has any abdominal pain, is no longer sick, and has identified the food triggers in her life. This seven-year-old no longer even chooses to eat the foods she now knows were making her sick.

There's no doubt that following the D.E.N.T.™ Program helps the person doing it, but it can also help their whole family.

YOU HAVE THE POWER

In your day-to-day life, you might believe—like too many of us—that you don't have the power to change things, that you are a victim of circumstances. You may believe that your genes determine your health and your destiny, but this fifty-year-old belief that our genetics determine our destiny is simply not true.

You Are In Control of Your Choices

How motivated are you to make changes?

My suggestion is that you look in the mirror.

Ask yourself:

- *How is my health?*
- *Am I happy?*
- *Do I feel strong?*
- *How energetic do I feel?*
- *How productive am I?*
- *What kind of choices do I make in my life every day?*

If the answers are not as positive as you would like them to be, then you need to ask yourself: *What am I willing to change?*

You need to seek education in order to empower yourself to make the right changes. There is so much information on the internet, and much of it is good, but it can be complicated and confusing.

You can look in the mirror and decide to change, and then you can seek information and education in order to empower yourself. Realize that the change you seek is difficult for most people to do on their own.

You can benefit from multiple kinds of support, such as:

- Coaching
- Mentoring
- Community

It's really difficult to make these changes all by yourself. This is why I have created the D.E.N.T.™ Program, which involves individual and group education, coaching, mentoring, and community support to empower you to be successful in restoring and optimizing your health.

Realize you have the power:

- You have the power to make the choice to change.

- You have the power to seek those who will be supportive.

- You have the power to ask your support system, the people in your life—your family, your partner, even your children—to be involved in the changes that are needing to happen.

You are more in control of your choices than you think. It starts with you. We are all familiar with the saying: *Your life depends on it.* Well, cross out the *it* and change it to YOU, because Your Life Depends On You!

Be responsible to yourself. Look in the mirror and ask yourself what you're willing to do.

Change can be easier and more successful when done in community. People who make an effort to lose weight aren't just helping themselves, they may be helping others too. A study done through the University of Connecticut tracked the weight loss progress of 130 couples over six months. The researchers found that when one member of a couple commits to losing weight, the chances were good the other partner would lose some weight too, even if they were not actively participating in a weight loss intervention.

In the study, approximately one-third of the untreated partners lost 3 percent or more of their initial body weight after six months, despite not participating in any active intervention. A 3 percent loss of body weight is considered a measurable health benefit.

The study's lead investigator, UConn Professor Amy Gorin, calls it a "ripple effect."

"When one person changes their behavior, the people around them change," says Gorin, a behavioral psychologist. "Whether the patient works with their healthcare provider, joins a community-based lifestyle approach, or tries to lose weight on their own, their new healthy behaviors can benefit others in their lives."[4]

You Can Do It

Once you've decided to change and have started taking steps in that direction, you can achieve your health goals. It's going to take time; things do not change overnight. But again, you need to seek education, community, and support.

With these three aspects firmly shoring up your resolve and action, modify your environment one step at a time. Then, you will start to heal. Your barriers will start to

---

4   Poitras, C. "Scientists Identify Weight Loss Ripple Effect." *UConn Today*. February 1, 2018. today.uconn.edu/2018/02/weight-loss-ripple-effect-helps-others/

heal. The information that you're feeding your genes, the information you're feeding your immune system, the information that you're feeding your microbiome will start to strengthen your body and make your fort stronger, your soldiers stronger, and therefore, your overall health will improve.

Life Can Be Better

Laurie is fifty-seven years old. She has suffered with anxiety and depression since she was thirty-five. She has had multiple hospitalizations and has a history of requiring electroconvulsive therapy to help bring her out of horrible anxiety and depression. Her original medical symptoms questionnaire score was ninety-five.

Laurie also complained of chronic fatigue and headaches. She's been diagnosed with hypothyroidism. She has sleep apnea, which means she needs to sleep with a machine that blows pressure into the back of her throat so she doesn't stop breathing episodically through the night. She has chronic, debilitating back pain and osteoarthritis. She has colitis with explosive diarrhea intermittently throughout her day. She has memory problems and struggles with obesity.

When she first came to me, she had already been working for six months on a diet to lose weight, and she had been successful in losing fifty-one pounds, but she still had essentially all her symptoms. She, too, commenced our D.E.N.T.™ Program.

Laurie undertook the diet and then the detox—the three-week elimination diet, in which you eliminate all the major foods that are triggers in the Standard American Diet.

Notice how the acronym for *Standard American Diet* is SAD?

Then she systematically re-challenged the different categories of foods, in order to identify what her food triggers are.

I saw her six weeks after completing the detox. She no longer has any diarrhea and her colitis has resolved. Her pain is so much improved that she's been able to go the gym and start exercising regularly. Her energy has improved, and her medical symptoms questionnaire has improved to score of thirty-three; not quite less than thirty yet, but she's getting there. She is excited, she is empowered, and she is hopeful.

Even within six weeks, someone can make these little changes in life, and life can be *significantly* better within a relatively short amount of time. This doesn't mean she's completely done on her path, and not everything is improved yet. But again, she is excited, she is empowered, and she is hopeful.

IT'S A JOURNEY RATHER THAN A DESTINATION

This is so important for people to understand: Who you are today is not who you were five or ten years ago. We are all changing, all the time. If you want to empower yourself and change your life and your future, you must realize that optimal health is a journey, not a destination, and it's going to happen one step at a time.

Your Health Won't Change Overnight

Life is a journey and each person's journey is unique. My journey started with watching my parents age, and for more than thirty years, it has led me to a passion for health and learning everything I can to keep my environment clean so that I do not go down the path of my genetics. I am the fifth of six children, and my mother didn't get married until she was thirty. I was in my late teens when I was watching my parents start to age.

My mother began losing her memory in her mid-to-late fifties. By the time she was in her early seventies, she was no longer driving. She had developed Alzheimer's dementia. I watched, from a relatively young age, as my mother lost her mind to the degree that she was gone from us before she ever physically died. I can remember like it was yesterday visiting my mom in the hospital when she was in her seventies; she and I were having such a nice visit and her lunch was brought in, so I got in her hospital bed with her and began to feed her. We were laughing, and I felt like we were connecting as if I was her little girl again.

But during this special moment, my mom turned to me and looked so confused and asked me in a hesitant voice, "What is your name? Who are you?"

My mom passed away at eighty-six years old, not able to move or communicate in any way, a vegetable in a bed.

I decided a long time ago to try to do everything I could to escape my genetics because I did not want to end up like my mom. I am currently fifty-five years old, and I have no memory problems. What I eat and how I live my life today are so different than when I was twenty or twenty-five, and it has been a journey of ups and downs and slow changes.

I can remember the first time I did a detox.

There were certain lines I drew in the sand, for example: *I will not stop putting honey and cream in my coffee. How bad can this one beverage be for me?*

After a few years of stopping the tea and coffee, I felt better, but still not as optimal as I would have liked. After learning more about the immune system and my own individual sensitivities, I am now completely caffeine and dairy free. I am also gluten free and try to follow a ketogenic lifestyle.

I live my life this way because I know that if I don't, I get sick. I didn't change my habits overnight. There have been many times when I struggled over giving things up and had to learn over and over that when I ingest even a little of these items, they make me sick.

The bottom line is that everyone makes a choice. We realize that who we are today and who we're going to be next month are not the same. Every day, I try to make choices to be healthier.

As an example, recently I realized my life had gotten out of balance and that I have not been taking time to exercise enough.

I looked in the mirror and asked myself what I was going to do to change this negative pattern that I had created?

I decided to change my schedule so that I could get back to the gym on Thursdays and go either to a yoga class or for a hike each Tuesday. These are changes I made in my lifestyle. The point I want to make here is that we evolve, and as long as we keep looking in the mirror, we're going to keep making the right changes that we need.

One Step at a Time

The D.E.N.T.™ Program that I have created to help you restore your health and put a dent in your chronic conditions is meant to help you focus on one facet of your life and one change or improvement at a time. As I have explained, we start with the Rainbow Diet concepts and then everyone puts themselves through a three-week detox or elimination diet in order to cleanse their system and to systematically identify their own individual food sensitivities.

Once the Diet is established, there is also education and coaching regarding Exercise, Nutrition, and self-Treatment.

In order to empower you, we emphasize that this is a step-by-step process, and help you go through the steps of the process one at a time at a pace that is personalized to your goals.

When you participate in the D.E.N.T.™ Program, you become part of a group who work through each step, one at a time.

Again, we start out with a rainbow diet concept. We help people who are eating more processed foods learn how to increase the color in their diet — by eating a greater variety of fruits and vegetables — and to decrease grains and so forth.

The next step, when you're ready — and this would be on your timeline, typically — is to do the elimination diet, or what I call the *Detox Plus Program*.

We also teach you about another pillar of health, *exercise and fitness*. There are a lot of myths about exercise, for instance: You need to exercise for hours in order to be optimally healthy. This is not true, so we teach you how to optimize your exercise and break through the myth.

We then educate people about how to *optimize their Nutrition*. Sometimes this is through supplements, but particularly, it's through your diet.

Then another step is to address *self-Treatment*, like meditation or a daily practice to reduce your stress, balance your stress levels, and reduce your cortisol, which is your stress hormone.

You'll notice there's one step at a time, one piece of information at a time, in order to help you step on the journey to restore and optimize your own health and be empowered.

Benefits Are Constant

Time and time again, the patients who come to our program report and give testimonials on our website that they feel better, they have more energy, they are thinking more clearly, and their brain fog is gone. They are actually less hungry and feel more fulfilled after eating. They feel joy and fulfillment after eating because they are eating *real* food, with *real* color, with *real* phytonutrients in it, and it is delicious! Most people think that the food is going to be boring, not delicious, and they're not going to like it. But every day, patients tell us they feel so much better after eating good food.

Luba, for example, is a patient who lost fifteen pounds within the first three weeks of changing to the rainbow diet. She had arthritis in her knee and after just three weeks, it was better. She said she smiled more, had more energy, and could think better. Luba's video testimonial is on my website discoverhealthfmc.com.

Knowing how well you can feel will help you stop reaching for the foods that you crave. The bad foods will lose their appeal because you know how unwell the bad foods make you feel. This helps you stay on the road and feel constantly empowered to be healthier on a daily basis.

I first started seeing Doctor Murray for chronic pain related to an injury in 2005. I was a very active runner before the injury and had not run in over eighteen months. I was unable to sit for more than thirty minutes without severe leg and back pain. It had gotten to the point of severely affecting my physical and mental well-being. Other doctors and physical therapy provided temporary relief that was never long-lasting.

Through the use of conservative treatments, manipulations, and prolotherapy, Dr. Murray had me back to running within a few months and on a continued plan to full health. I continue to see Dr. Murray for regular adjustments and I appreciate her holistic and whole-body approach to my wellness. I feel that Trish really takes the time to really listen to her patients to work together on treatments that make sense for each individual. My wife and one of my children have also seen her. I would recommend her to anyone.

~ Paul Kirsch

CHAPTER THREE

Food Is Information

*The most difficult thing had been the decision to act,
the rest was merely tenacity — and the fears were paper
tigers. . . . One could really act to change and control one's
life; and the procedure, the process, was its own reward.*
~ Robyn Davidson, *Tracks*

YOUR FOOD CHOICES CAN LEAD TOWARD EITHER HEALTH OR ILLNESS

We put food in our mouths so many times each day without really thinking about the fact that food is information. Food is full of chemicals, and it can be good information — such as vitamins, minerals, phytonutrients, and antioxidants — or it can potentially be poison. What I am hoping to help you realize is that every bite of food you take provides your body and mind with either good health-promoting information or bad disease-promoting information. Once you realize this and understand how important it is to your health and your overall well-being, you will be on your way to restoring and optimizing your own health.

Eat the Rainbow

I've mentioned the Rainbow Concept before. What I mean by this is that eating a variety of colors of fruits and vegetables will give you a broad diversity of nutrients. Consider the colors of the rainbow: red, orange, yellow, green, blue, and purple.

Can you think of natural foods that match each color?

It's easiest to see these in fruits and vegetables.

Why do foods have these different colors?

Our maker created plants in different colors as indicators of the compounds they contain. For example, *antioxidants* are important compounds for our health because they neutralize free radicals. Free radicals are charged particles that are formed when our body attempts to detoxify chemicals or waste products. These positively charged free radicals are dangerous to our tissues and cause degeneration and damage. Antioxidants are negatively charged particles that bind with free radicals to neutralize them and stop them from causing damage. *Carotenoids* are full of antioxidants and come from red, orange, and yellow plants. *Resveratrol* comes from purple foods, such as dark red grapes, and is an anti-inflammatory, antioxidant, and anti-aging nutrient.

Here is a list of some foods from each color and their health benefits:

Yellow foods like pineapple, summer squash, lemons, and corn contain the nutrients zeaxanthin, flavonoids, lycopene, potassium, vitamin C, and beta-carotene, which is a form of vitamin A.

Orange foods like butternut squash, carrots, cantaloupe, and sweet potatoes share similar nutrients to yellow fruits and vegetables. These nutrients help lower cholesterol, decrease risk of cancer, promote collagen formation for healthy joints, and decrease damaging free radicals.

Green foods like asparagus, avocados, kiwi, broccoli, leeks, and spinach contain the nutrients chlorophyll, lutein, calcium, folate, vitamin C, fiber, and beta-carotene. These nutrients support optimal detoxification, lower blood pressure, normalize digestion, support good vision, and boost the immune system.

Red foods like beets, cherries, cranberries, radishes, rhubarb, and pomegranates contain the nutrients lycopene, quercetin, and hesperidin. These nutrients can help with lung and breathing problems, protect DNA from damage, and decrease risk of prostate cancer.

Blue and Purple foods like blueberries, eggplant, purple potatoes, plums, and grapes contain the nutrients resveratrol, flavonoids, quercetin, vitamin C, fiber, and zeaxanthin. These nutrients slow the aging process, decrease inflammation, protect and strengthen the lining of arteries, and decrease toxic stress.

Plants provide us with so many nutrients. You are probably familiar with vitamins, like A, B, C, D, and E, as well as minerals, like zinc, selenium, and magnesium. These are all extremely important to health, but there's a whole other category, called *phytonutrients. Phyto-* is the prefix meaning "plant," and -*nutrient,* of course, speaks for itself. Phytonutrients or phytochemicals are produced by plants in order to protect them from damaging agents in their environment, such as germs, molds, pollution, and toxins. They also are responsible for the color, flavor, and smell of a plant. There are over 25,000 different phytonutrients that come from plants, and these protective chemicals can protect us from environmental dangers in the same way they protect the plant.

With all this being said, it should be clear why we need to eat a primarily plant-based diet full of a rainbow variety of colors. As a rule of thumb, you should eat at least one serving of every color of the rainbow every forty-eight hours.

Foods You Eat Every Day Could Be Causing Disruption

How do you feel after you eat a meal?

It's easy to notice or be mindful of what you've eaten when it makes you feel ill. Other times you might be mindful because you feel better. Most days, however, most of us mindlessly put food in our mouths.

Becoming mindful of what you eat is another way to pay attention to your health. There may be foods that you are eating every day that cause disruption to the protective barriers we discussed in earlier chapters: your skin, intestinal wall, or even your blood-brain barrier. Foods that are damaging or destructive to these different barriers are the most common environmental triggers that can throw your immune system off balance.

Some of the most inflammatory foods are:

- Dairy, including fermented or cultured dairy, such as yogurt
- Gluten
- Soy
- Alcohol
- Sugar

These culprits can cause the iceberg of inflammation and autoimmunity that needs to be melted. The barrier breakdown typically begins in the gut where the intestinal lining becomes leaky. Once foreign or damaging chemicals or particles leak through the intestinal lining, they then can travel through the bloodstream to damage other barriers, such as your blood-brain barrier, and cause more neurological problems.

Now, you may be thinking: *But I don't have gut concerns. I typically don't have problems related to my gastrointestinal system.*

I want you to remember that three things must be present to develop inflammation and autoimmunity:

1. Genetic susceptibility
2. Barrier dysfunction
3. Environmental triggers

Your genetic susceptibilities put you at a level of risk. For example, if you're at risk for nonceliac gluten sensitivity, then gluten-containing foods are going to disrupt your barriers. This typically is a disruption of your intestinal lining but can also lead to a disruption of your blood-brain barrier. You may not present with gut-related symptoms, but you may present with more neurological-related symptoms, such as anxiety, depression, brain fog, or cognitive decline.

If the foods you are eating or the damaging chemicals you are exposed to on a daily basis are breaking down your gut barrier, this can be the root cause of your chronic dis-ease processes. They can irritate your immune system and travel in your body to break down other protective barriers. It can be the main reason why you have developed a large, under-the-surface iceberg of inflammation and immune system hypersensitivity that will present based on your genetic susceptibility.

Sugar Is Your Enemy; Fat Is Not

We are living in an era of epidemic diabetes, obesity, and cognitive decline or Alzheimer's disease rates. You must understand that sugar is your enemy. Sugar is pro-inflammatory and a neurotoxin. It is common knowledge that sugar causes diabetes, but studies have shown that the higher the blood sugar, the smaller the brain and that an increased carbohydrate or sugar-filled diet increases risk of dementia by 89 percent.[5]

Grains are a category of food that also fuels the high carbohydrate, sugar-filled diet.

---

5   Perlmutter, D. "Rethinking Dietary Approaches for Brain Health." Alternative and Complimentary Therapies. (20:2) April 10, 2014. doi.org/10.1089/act.2014.20206.
    Roberts, R. "Relative Intake of Macronutrients Impacts Risk of Mild Cognitive Impairment or Dementia" Journal of Alzheimer's Disease (32:2) 2012. 329–339.

Some examples of grains or grain products are:

- Pasta
- Bread
- Rice
- Cereal

From the moment you take grains and grain products into your mouth and start the digestive process, they are converted to glucose. Glucose is sugar. The average American eats six or seven servings of grain *every day*. That's an enormous amount of sugar. If you start out your morning with a bowl of cereal and a piece of toast, you've just eaten two or three servings already.

Then, the typical lunch consists of a sandwich and a snack, such as pretzels, which is at least three more servings of grain. We then are hungry a few hours later and reach for a muffin or chips, and then dinner always typically includes a grain or grain product, such as rice or pasta. This all adds up to as many as six to eight servings of grain per day, and all of it gets converted to glucose.

I suggest you count for yourself: How many servings of grains do you eat in a typical day?

If you're like most people, you're eating too many and producing too much sugar.

I recommend you eat only one or two servings of grains per day, period.

Now, I get it — grains have been a staple in your diet for a long time and they help to fill you up, so you are wondering what you will substitute for them.

Well, the whole reason we eat is to give ourselves fuel for energy. Calories are the way we measure the amount of fuel we are providing our bodies at any given meal. This is why grains and carbohydrates have been the base of our meals because they have less calories than fats do. For example, each gram of carbohydrate provides four calories of energy and each gram of protein also provides four calories of energy; but, each gram of fat provides nine calories of energy. Fat has nearly twice as many calories as carbohydrates or protein and this is why we have been taught to avoid fats. But, you need to understand that nine calories from the same amount of food will actually sustain you and your energy level longer than four calories will. This is why you typically are hungry again within a few hours of eating a high-carbohydrate meal.

Over the last fifty years, we have been taught that fat is bad:

Low fat, no fat, don't give me any fat because I'm going to get fat!

Well, that's wrong. That's incorrect information.

You don't want to eat *bad* fats: Trans fats and hydrogenated fats are bad for you. Processed foods and vegetable oils are bad for you.

Good fats are filling, energy sustaining, feed your brain, which is made up of 60 percent fat, and improve immune system function.

Below is a list of good fats for you to eat:

- Extra virgin olive oil
- Olives
- Coconut oil and coconut milk
- Avocados
- Nuts
- Seeds

The bottom line here is to avoid grains. It's not that everyone should avoid grains altogether; instead, limit the number of servings you eat each day to one or two and increase your servings of health-promoting fats. These simple changes sustained over time will help you lose weight, decrease your sugar levels, quiet your inflammation, and promote optimal energy and brain function.

WE ARE ALL DIFFERENT

Each individual is different. We all know that. People look different, act different, and react differently. This is obvious.

How does individual difference apply to food and nutrition?

What one person is going to be sensitive to or allergic to is going to be very different compared to the next person.

One Person's Nutrient Is Another Person's Poison

Food can be either healthful or harmful to you. It depends to some degree on whether you have food allergies or sensitivities. A *food allergy* causes a dramatic reaction to the skin, breathing, or digestion. For example, a child with a peanut allergy who accidentally eats one might immediately break out in a rash, or possibly have a horrible reaction like anaphylactic shock. An allergic reaction is obvious. A child with a peanut allergy cannot eat peanuts, ever. In some cases, the allergy can be so severe that simply being around peanuts can cause a reaction. A true food allergy is one type of reaction from your immune system; it is an *IgE antibody reaction*.

A subtler reaction is called a *food sensitivity*. Symptoms of food sensitivities do not always appear immediately. They can develop anywhere from moments to up to seventy-two hours later. So, you may not notice a negative reaction for two to three days after you eat gluten, for example. And due to the delayed reaction, it is difficult to identify which specific foods are the culprit. As a result, you may be eating foods you are sensitive to every day and your immune system is constantly irritated. Food sensitivities result in your immune system from a different reaction, called an *IgG antibody reaction*.

The point is that you may have to eat differently from another person if you have a food allergy or a food sensitivity. Also, a food sensitivity may be harder to detect because it may take days to present itself. If you are eating foods you have a sensitivity to every day, then your immune system is irritated and developing inflammation constantly and you feel lousy. For many people, if *lousy* is the baseline and they do not know any different, then identifying food sensitivities and eliminating them from the day-to-day menu can help them feel better.

The Elimination Concept Can Identify Your Triggers

The good news is that you can identify your food sensitivities or triggers.

Here is a more complete list of foods that are common triggers, and therefore to be avoided, in the Standard American Diet (SAD):

- Gluten, which is in wheat, barley, and rye
- Dairy
- Peanuts
- Corn
- Eggs
- Shellfish
- Soy
- Nightshades—tomatoes, potatoes, eggplant, and peppers

Anyone can empower themselves to identify their own food sensitivities by doing a comprehensive elimination diet. This is done by eliminating all the foods listed above for three weeks or twenty-one days. This will allow your body to cleanse itself of all triggers and quiet your immune system.

YOU HAVE THE POWER TO KNOW WHAT'S GOOD FOR YOU AND WHAT'S NOT

In order to educate and support people to implement a comprehensive elimination diet, I have created a course I call the *Detox Plus Program*. This course consists of a guidebook and five video-based supportive lectures to explain the process one step at a time.

You Can Do Anything for Twenty-One Days

The first thing that just about everyone says to me when I suggest they consider doing the Detox Plus Program or the comprehensive elimination diet is: *You've got to be kidding me! How will I give up all these different foods, and what will I eat?*

Another question people ask me is: *How can I do it for that long?*

I explain to people that they are not going to start this immediately.

This is a process that you must prepare for. The Detox Plus Program provides you with the education and support you need to be successful. It is a five- to six-week program available on my website (discoverhealthfmc. com). There you'll find a guidebook you can print out, as well as five talks you can listen to. I support you to take it one step at a time.

You are going to learn about it, think it over, and then look at your calendar and ask yourself: *When can I schedule focusing on my health for the twenty-one days?*

If you look at the whole program all at once, it seems overwhelming.

But if you take your time and read through the material a few times, I'm sure it will make sense and you'll realize you can do this. You need to take the time to become familiar with it and then set your mind to it. Once you set your mind to it, there will be no holding you back.

By the end of the twenty-one days, everyone who has done the program comes to me and says, "Trish, I have not felt this good in the last ten years, and I don't want to stop doing this!"

I tell them that is fine! You can continue the elimination diet for as long as you like because it is a healthy way of eating. It is anti-inflammatory and healing. The volume of food or the number of calories one eats on this program is not limited; only the choice of the food items is limited or restricted. But, I also warn people not to miss out on the *Plus* portion of the program by not re-challenging the different categories of food triggers properly.

How to Systematically Re-Challenge

The next step after the Detox is the Plus step. During this step, you will re-challenge each category of eliminated foods systematically to identify which are your individual triggers.

I tell every patient that at the end of the twenty-one days, on day twenty-two, you do not want to say:

Woohoo! Now, I can go out and have a pizza and a beer because I survived the detox!

If you do that, you will have lost the opportunity to systematically re-challenge the different categories or individual foods. You will not be able to empower yourself by absolutely identifying which foods are your individual triggers.

Instead, the next step is to slowly add foods back into your menu and gauge how they make you feel. In this manner, you will be able to identify your own sensitivities, and therefore avoid those foods to make your immune system balanced and healthy. You can melt the iceberg that has been growing. You can stop eating the triggers that have been irritating your immune system, causing your inflammation, and making you feel lousy.

To initiate the re-challenge correctly, on day twenty-two, pick the individual food or category of food that you are missing the most.

If a patient says to me, "Trish, I've got to have a piece of cheese," or, "I've got to have a glass of milk," I say to them, "Re-challenge dairy first."

On day one of re-challenging, eat one to two servings of that food, such as dairy.

Days two and three, up to seventy-two hours, you're going to eat that food again. Remember, a food sensitivity can present itself anywhere up to three days.

However, if you have a negative reaction right after eating your test food on day one, then obviously don't continue to eat it and feel horrible. Realize right away that that is a food trigger for you. Get it back off your menu and wait until you're feeling well again until you move onto the second category you're going to re-challenge.

If you eat the test food on day one, and you feel fine, you eat it on day two, and wait, and eat it on day three. If for all seventy-two hours—three days—you have not had any negative reactions, then you can be clear that that category of food is not your trigger, and you can put it back in your regular daily diet confidently. Then you systematically keep re-challenging each one of the food categories, such as peanuts, eggs, soy, and so on; until you identify each and every one of your food sensitivities and you are clear on them.

What to Do Once You've Identified Your Triggers

What is the next step?

Continue for another month to eliminate only the categories or the individual foods that you identified that caused you problems. At the end of that month, you can re-challenge those different categories or items again, following the seventy-two–hour/three-day process. If you still find yourself sensitive to all of them, or only some of them, then continue to eliminate the ones that cause a negative response for another month. You notice you can keep cycling this concept, because once you understand this concept, you can always apply it over and over again.

The thing that I also want you to understand is that over time, your leaky gut may heal. The mucous membranes, the cilia, the tight junctions between the cells may heal. So, you may not be sensitive to the different foods forever. You may need to avoid them only for the amount of time it takes for the gut to heal. You may not notice the same negative response. However, some of us are not so lucky, and we may be sensitive to these foods forever. For example, I am gluten-sensitive, dairy-sensitive, and caffeine-sensitive. I have been for six or seven years. No matter how much time goes by, when I re-challenge these items, they cause a problem. I simply continue to avoid them, and that keeps my immune system and me healthy.

Once you've identified your triggers, you want to continue to avoid them, but you could keep re-challenging them, let's say, once every few months. Over time, you may notice that these sensitivities will improve, but for others, you may never notice that. That sensitivity may be permanent.

There are some blood tests available that can identify a person's food sensitivities, but these tests are not standardized. From test to test, there is no laboratory standardization. The gold-standard test for anyone to identify their food triggers is the comprehensive elimination diet, or what I call the *Detox Plus Program*. Also, I have seen many times that a person spends hundreds of dollars to have a blood test done to identify their food sensitivities and the results come back stating they are sensitive to most every food. This result typically occurs because of the underlying leaky gut that is present. I have learned from experience that to have clients put themselves through the Detox Plus Program to initiate the healing of their gut lining and quiet their inflammation and change their lifestyle is a much more empowering path.

For more details about the Detox Plus Program, see the Conclusion and Next Steps sections of this book.

Time Heals

Once you have identified your food environmental triggers, your leaky gut is most likely going to heal. The tight junctions between the epithelial cells that make up the wall or barrier that keeps your gut healthy will become strong again. They'll keep the waste products inside the hose of your digestive tract and safely guide them out of your body.

Your immune system is going to be healthier because it won't be constantly responding to triggers. Your police and your military are going to be able to rest, and your iceberg will melt. This process is extremely empowering for people because once you understand the elimination concept and process, then you can apply it repeatedly and over time, you are going to restore and optimize your own health!

The reason we first came to Discover Health was because we feel that today's Western medicine does not make anybody healthy. It didn't make us healthy. We sought to help ourselves, but there was still something missing. We raise our own food and live mostly farm to table, but there was still something missing. When my husband saw the advertisement in the paper for Trish Murray's free talk we thought we'd try it out. My husband Dan saw it first, and we're very glad we came.

Dr. Murray has taught us about nutrition and diet, which has been very helpful versus trying to change numbers on a chart with a prescription drug, and I (Dan) like that.

I (Merrily) found out things I know I never would have found out going to a traditional Western doctor. All my problems, Trish Murray said from the get-go were from allergies. And I did not realize how bad they were until I had testing done, even after I did the detox diet. (We had done detox diets in the past.) From the testing, I learned I was allergic to things I was eating a lot of; if not eating the most of! And taking those things out of my diet was a big improvement!

For anybody who is at their wits' end about not feeling good or don't know what feeling good is, try Discover Health Functional Medicine Center and learn how much changing your diet and other lifestyle things can help!

~ Merrily and Dan Brennon

CHAPTER FOUR

Stress

If you change your perception, you can change your emotion, and this can lead to new ideas.
~ Edward de Bono

WE LIVE IN A STRESSFUL WORLD

I don't think I need to tell anybody or prove to anyone that we live in a stressful world. Stress is another environmental trigger that can lead to inflammation and autoimmunity. It can lead to imbalance in multiple systems of your body—particularly your immune system—and lead down the path of inflammation, autoimmunity, and chronic dis-ease.

You Can't Avoid Stress

None of us can avoid stress. Over the last fifty years or more, stress has increased in the average person's world. Fifty years ago, if a couple married and had children, typically one of them could have stayed home to care for the family and the home. Today, that's just not so. With financial stresses, both adults typically need to work outside the home, which makes time management more stressful. Let's say five days a week, eight hours a day you're at work, and then you go home and take care of the household. Even if you thoroughly enjoy your job, this change has significantly increased daily responsibilities and stress levels.

Our children's lives have become more stressful. Children today typically don't go outside and play like we did forty or fifty years ago. They are scheduled all the time: to go to sports practices, take an art or dance class, or attend a club or community group.

On top of these demands, add the financial concerns of the continual rise in inflation, along with the fact that the typical hourly wage today without a college degree does not sustain a family comfortably.

Beyond this, you have relationships that you want to maintain, such as the relationship with your spouse, family, and friends. All these relationships take effort and time to nurture and maintain.

Add these stressors together, and we can all see it's impossible to avoid the stress of our era.

You can't avoid stress, but you have the power to modify and control your choices and your perception of the different struggles and challenges in your life.

Not All Stress Is Bad

Stress is an awesome motivator. If you didn't have *any* stress in your life, you wouldn't reach the levels you do and most likely would not be motivated or pushed to reach your full potential. Some of the most famous people in the world have faced extreme failures and challenges in their lives.

Those failures and challenges caused them to reach their full potential and become famous with the optimally fulfilling lives they led:

- Michael Jordan, one of the most famous professional basketball players in the world, wasn't chosen for the varsity team in his sophomore year of high school. Rather than let that stop him, he tried even harder to make varsity the next year and was successful.

- Abraham Lincoln lost a number of elections and experienced a couple business failures before he was elected president.

- Stephen King, one of the most famous authors of thriller fiction novels, had thirty rejections before *Carrie* was accepted for publication. It eventually was not only a best-selling novel, but a blockbuster movie.

- Steven Spielberg, one of the most famous producers of blockbuster films, was denied admittance to University of Southern California's movie and theater college before he went on to direct over fifty films and win three Oscars.

These are perfect examples that not all stress is bad.

You can view negative outcomes as simple failures, or you can view them as motivators and challengers to push you beyond what you ever thought was possible.

Perception

When you view an event or circumstance as stressful, if you focus on negative emotions—such as irritation, frustration, helplessness, or hopelessness—then these emotions affect your perception. With a negative perception, you can't be motivated. Your perception keeps you back and makes you feel that everything is a struggle.

Negative perception increases your stress. Instead of viewing difficult times from a place of negativity and frustration, view stresses and struggles from a place of gratitude for the way those struggling times push you.

If you do this, you'll notice your times of hardship will push you to more success.

If you always come from a place of negativity and negative emotions, this sets up a patterned response in your being in your physiology, biochemical pathways, nervous system, hormonal balance, and your gut. For example, increased negative thinking and stress will affect your ability to digest food properly and can be a root cause for leaky gut. If you are always coming at stress from a negative place and your nervous system is always stressed out, then your cortisol level is always going to be elevated.

Increased levels of cortisol, your primary stress hormone, will also block the production of appropriate amounts of thyroid hormone and can be a root cause of hypothyroidism. Elevated cortisol levels also block the production of healthy neurotransmitters like serotonin. Serotonin is a major neurotransmitter produced primarily in your gut. It helps stabilize mood and optimizes digestion as well as sleep. Many people with depression, for example, are put on a category of antidepressant medication called *selective serotonin reuptake inhibitors*. These medications try to affect a person's physiology to increase the serotonin levels in their bloodstream. A functional medicine approach realizes that stress and resulting elevated cortisol are the root causes for low levels of serotonin and your depression. Your treatment plan should include stress-management techniques to get to the root cause of the problem, rather than more and more prescription medications.

And each of the different physiologic effects of increased stress and cortisol can act like dominoes in a series of systemic dysfunctions. For example, if increased stress leads to less stomach acid, and less stomach acid leads to poor digestion, and poor digestion sets you up for leaky gut, then based on what we explained earlier, more undigested particles are going to leak through your intestinal wall and irritate your immune system.

Your immune system is then going to get irritated by more and more foreign stranger dangers and all these imbalances lead to:

- Inflammation
- Hypersensitivity
- Autoimmune disease
- Chronic disease

YOUR PERCEPTION DRIVES YOUR STRESS LEVEL

There are environmental triggers in your life that put you at risk for inflammation, autoimmunity, and chronic disease. Your ability to modify your environmental triggers and to change your perception of the challenges in your life are the answers to preventing or reversing your chronic disease. *This is the number-one thing I want you to learn from this book.*

We Are Emotional Beings

We think of ourselves as rational, cognitive beings, but we are not. We are emotional beings first and rational beings second. Your attention, perception, memory, logical reasoning, and rational decision-making abilities are secondary to your emotions.

This is because the regions of our brain that are fundamental to our mood and emotions are in the oldest and most primordial areas of our brain. These fundamental regions are called the *limbic system*. The limbic system is the major primordial brain network underpinning our mood and our emotions. It is a network of regions that include the hypothalamus, hippocampus, and amygdala. These regions of our brain work together to make sense of our world. For example, the hypothalamus modulates hormones associated with mood and survival. The hippocampus reminds us of which behaviors led to outcomes that are consistent with our present mood or emotional state. And the amygdala attaches emotional significance to present events and to our memories. This region regulates biological functions in conjunction with our mood, such as increased heart rate or sweating triggered by feeling flustered or irritated.

Your emotions are central to your experience of stress. Your perception of a stimulus as a threat is what causes stress. Anger and negative emotions provide the fuel for our stress. Stress is truly emotional dis-ease.

Think back to a stressful situation when there were other people around you experiencing the same stress:

- How did you respond?
- How did others?
- Did everyone have the same reaction?

You may have responded more emotionally than the next person, or another person may have responded more emotionally than you. I'm sure everyone has been in a situation where they've noted with surprise that they responded with less of a stressful charge to a situation than another person.

We Act Before We Think

When you are upset, let's say, if you're fighting with your spouse or you're frustrated with your child, it's harder to think straight. Your emotional mind takes over and drowns out our more reasonable or rational thoughts. In emotionally charged situations like this, it is completely unproductive to try and resolve the engagement until you can walk away and calm down enough to begin processing the situation with the rational areas of your brain.

You've probably had the experience of walking away from a situation in which you argued with someone you love, and you've said to yourself: *I can't believe I said that. I can't believe I did that.*

When you are in an emotionally charged or threatening situation, your nervous system automatically reacts with a fight-or-flight response. This fight-or-flight response is activated in your sympathetic nervous system and bypasses your conscious, cognitive processing areas of your brain. This is why when you feel threatened, you react first and think about your actions later. In these situations, your emotions can control you, and you are not able to think straight or process rationally until you walk away and calm down.

You Can't Think Yourself Down

Again, when your negative emotions are up and you are in an emotionally charged state, you cannot think yourself down. We've given the example of a one-time argument, and the example of doing or saying things that we can't imagine we would ever do.

But what if you have constant emotional distress, and your brain has become accustomed to this pattern as normal?

If you live in a constant state of feeling threatened or always perceive the world from negative emotions — such as fear, anger, frustration, or irritation — then this is the pattern that is going to be established and become hardwired in your system. This is of great concern because once it's a pattern, it's going to run your nervous system. Once it's running your nervous system, this pattern will affect other systems, such as your hormonal balance, your cardiovascular system, and your immune system. The constant pattern of stress response can lead to imbalance, dysfunction, and chronic disease. A pattern of chronic stress can also disrupt your life to the point that you feel paralyzed and cannot make productive decisions.

Connie is an elderly patient of mine. She and her husband bought a farm after they retired from their work lives in their early- to mid-sixties. They moved from the city up to a farm in the mountains of New Hampshire, and they loved their life on their farm. But about five years ago, the husband passed away.

Connie has downsized the farm, but she is still managing the animals and her farm by herself. She's developed chronic back pain. She already survived lung cancer once, but it is starting to rise up in her life again. She talks about how fearful, concerned, and frustrated she is with not being able to manage her life, but she also expresses that she feels paralyzed and unable to quiet herself enough to process her situation rationally so that she can make the right decisions and decide how she wants to live out the remaining years of her life.

This is why chronic stress is so dangerous. It can disrupt your body systems and cause dis-ease, but it also can establish a pattern in your life that keeps you from being able to process things well and can paralyze you.

None of us are immune to this danger. This can happen to anyone at any age; for example, a college student who is fearful and frustrated with their need to have the right friends, or to get the right grades, or to live up to peer pressure. They will feel anxious and depressed and not be able to be as productive as they would like. Until they can quiet their mind and their nervous system enough to be able to ask themselves what they truly want for themselves, they will continue to be confused, frustrated, and paralyzed. Or, consider a person in their forties who has a job and is in the peak of their adult life but is also faced with many financial demands with a mortgage for their home, taxes, children now in college, and is wanting to have some fun traveling. They may develop frustration, fear, and concern, and these perceptions of their challenges create the stressful charge to the situation and make it difficult for the mind to quiet enough to see the choices clearly. A person in their forties, in a job, in the peak of their life, tries to make financial decisions, but they're paralyzed by the same pattern of not looking at things in a positive way, or not being able to quiet their being enough to make the right financial decisions.

So, you can't think rationally when you're paralyzed by stress. If you find that you are feeling constant stress and perceiving your challenges negatively, then it is time for you to learn a new way of perceiving what life is handing you.

YOU HAVE THE POWER TO CHANGE YOUR OWN PERCEPTION

Education is power and I would like to empower you by teaching you how to modify your perceptions of the challenges in your life. You can perceive your challenges, struggles, and stresses differently. You can learn to see them more positively, as motivators, and in so doing, you can quiet your mind to make more clear decisions, and you can balance the multiple systems of your body and improve your physiology and biochemistry.

The Nervous System

We actually should say the *nervous systems,* plural, because there are multiple parts to the overall nervous system of your body:

1. There is the *central nervous system,* which is made up of your brain and your spinal cord.

2. There is the *peripheral nervous system,* which is made up of the nerves that branch off your spinal cord and go out into your arms, your fingers, your hands, your legs, your feet, and your toes. You touch the stove and it's hot; you sense that and respond by moving your hand away. This is also known as your *voluntary nervous system* because you can consciously control the movements of these muscles.

3. There is a third, very important part of your nervous system called the *autonomic nervous system,* or the *automatic nervous system.* This is also known as the *involuntary nervous system* because it governs things you can't consciously control, such as heart rate, body temperature, and digestive processes, such as salivation.

The autonomic nervous system has two parts:

1. The sympathetic nervous system
2. The parasympathetic nervous system

These two parts of the automatic nervous system must stay in balance.

The sympathetic nervous system is your *fight-or-flight* nervous system. If you are stressed, and you experience or perceive a stress as fearful, irritating, angering, or frustrating, you are going to have a fight-or-flight response.

Certain neurotransmitters and hormones—such as adrenaline, cortisol, and norepinephrine—are elevated when fight-or-flight is activated.

These chemicals cause:

- Increased heart rate
- Constriction of blood vessels
- Increase in your blood pressure

All these physiologic changes help move blood away from your organs to your muscles, so you can run away from or fight any threat coming at you.

The parasympathetic nervous system regulates and governs your organs, digestion, relaxation, libido, and sleep.

For example, your sex drive is not going to be in full gear when you're stressed out and frustrated all the time. Your parasympathetic nervous system, which innervates your gut, your liver, your spleen, your lungs, your heart, and yes, your sex organs, needs to be in balance with the sympathetic nervous system.

The physiologic effects of the parasympathetic nervous system include:

- Reduced heart rate
- Reduced blood pressure
- Improved digestion
- Increased libido or sex drive
- Relaxed breathing

These two nervous systems must be in balance. If you are always in a stressful situation and your sympathetic nervous system is always running the show, then you will always have high blood pressure, you'll always be in fight-or-flight response. Again, that's going to set off a pattern that sends you down the road toward hypersensitivity, hyperreactivity, and imbalance. And this is going to cause leaky gut and chronic inflammation, which many times is the root cause of the growth of the iceberg in your body that leads to chronic disease.

Change Your Perception and Change Your Patterns

In order to break the cycle of your chronic stress pattern of negative emotions, you need to learn how to balance your stress and come at it from a more positive place.

You need to change your patterns, and the biggest hurdle to this process is first realizing that you *can* change your patterns. Most of the patterns of our lives are stored in our subconscious.

You see, we all have a *subconscious mind* or a *subconscious being,* and a *conscious mind* or a *conscious being.* Our subconscious mind or being is a million times more powerful than our conscious mind or being. That is, until you bring to your conscious mind something that you want to change.

Once you bring it to your conscious mind, then your conscious mind is a million billion times more powerful than your subconscious mind, and you have the power to change beliefs, routines, and expectations of yourself.

You may become consciously aware that you are responding to the stresses in your life primarily from the emotions of:

- Anger
- Irritation
- Hopelessness
- Fear
- Helplessness

Once you consciously recognize this negative pattern of responding to or looking at challenges, then you can commit to changing the negative pattern. You can consciously work toward shifting your emotional perception of the challenges by emphasizing more positive emotions, such as:

- Gratitude
- Appreciation
- Compassion
- Thankfulness
- Praise

It is a simple solution, but it does require work — just because it's simple doesn't mean it's easy. It takes repetition and practice to shift your focus. When you make positive emotions the universal feeling or expression from your being, then you can see that your patterns, physiology, and biochemistry change and settle into a more positive response to life's challenges.

In order to explore these concepts further, I recommend watching a TED talk by Jill Bolte-Taylor. She is a neuroanatomist who had a stroke one day due to a blood clot the size of a golf ball in the left hemisphere of her brain. She's written a book about the experience called *My Stroke of Insight*. On the day of her stroke, her left hemisphere — which is the side of your brain that is responsible for all the details of our life, the emotional baggage, the part of your brain that makes you separate from everyone else—was quiet. Only the right side of her brain could function normally. The right side of the brain governs creativity. It's the part of your brain that connects you to all that is, everyone and everything. It is your loving, universal brain.

In her book and her TED talk, Jill Bolte-Taylor explains her amazing experience of feeling free from any emotional baggage, demands, or separateness. She explains that she felt euphoria, connection, peace, and oneness with the universe. She luckily survived her stroke and recovered. She decided to share with the world the lesson she learned that day: we can learn to quiet the detail-oriented, left side of our brain that keeps us focused on emotional baggage and separateness, and instead enhance the right side of our brain that connects us all as one and fills us with peace and harmony. She calls this "stepping to the right of your left hemisphere," to feel the same sense of oneness she did without having to experience a stroke. If we can all step to the right of our left hemisphere, let go of our emotional baggage, and connect to all that is, the universe will help us quiet our minds and change our perceptions in a positive way.

Tools to Help You

Now that you understand that stress is truly emotional un-ease or a negative perception toward the challenges in your life and that the answer to decreasing your stress requires changing your emotional response or perception, it should make sense that a prescription medication is not going to make this shift for you. We have been trained to believe that there is a pill for every ill and that simply taking our daily medications should make us feel better. But, this *pill for every ill* mentality must go if we are going to reverse our chronic disease conditions.

Instead, we must modify our environmental triggers and change our perceptions by stepping to the right of our left hemisphere. To do this, we must each develop a daily practice of spending five to ten minutes enhancing our parasympathetic nervous system and enhancing the right side of our brains. Below are some simple and straightforward exercises that you can start implementing today.

Start with your breathing:

1. Sit with your feet flat on the floor, in a comfortable position.

2. Close your eyes and take a deep breath.

3. To give your left brain something to do, count to 5 as you slowly inhale.

4. Exhale for a count to 7.

You'll notice that you're breathing out for longer than you're breathing in. That's because inhalation is more of a sympathetic nervous system exercise and exhalation is more of a relaxation, parasympathetic exercise. If you can breathe in for a count of five, and you breathe out for a count of seven, you're going to emphasize relaxation through your parasympathetic nervous system. Again, when you count in and you count out, you're giving your left brain something to do and keeping it occupied so that your physiology, your hormones, your mind, and your being can relax.

Once you are comfortable with the focused breathing, now add another step.

Bring in positive emotions while you're breathing:

1. Inhale for a count of 5, and think of something you are grateful for.

2. Exhale for a count of 7, and think of someone or something you have compassion for or are thankful for in your life.

You'll notice that by bringing in these positive emotions and emphasizing the parasympathetic nervous system, you are going to relax yourself and start shifting your physiology, your biochemistry, and your whole being.

You will start to feel lighter, more connected, and will start stepping to the right of your left hemisphere.

Once you have practiced adding positive emotions to your breathing and you feel comfortable with it, you may choose to add a positive affirmation to your practice.

Repeat positive affirmations:

1. On the inhale, focus on an affirmation that you would like to embrace, such as, "I am powerful and can modify my life for the better." Breathe in and say that affirmation.

2. Repeat the affirmation as you exhale.

These tools are most helpful when you use them every day. They are simple and straightforward, but in order to truly shift your patterns, you must make them a daily practice.

At least five to ten minutes most days of your life, you must practice some of these tools that allow you to:

*   Emphasize your positive emotions
*   Bring your sympathetic and parasympathetic nervous systems into better balance
*   Quiet your being so that you do not feel paralyzed by stress
*   Take control and modify your environmental triggers

I started coming to Discover Health about a year ago and Trish Murray, DO, had been recommended to me. So, I went in and had my first appointment, and we decided together that I would start with the D.E.N.T.™ curriculum. The three-week detox is pretty intense; however, the feedback it gives you is amazing! And when you really start feeling better, it's amazing what you can do. The energy I felt going through the detox, the information I learned about my body when the correct food is put in, the mental clarity was pretty amazing!

I also talked about neurofeedback with Trish and initiated this therapy and have done nine sessions so far. What an amazing process to go through! It's very simple. It's not intimidating. After my second session, I started sleeping through the night, which was amazing! It's changing my life with my anxiety, the way I feel and my ability to deal with it if things really arise and panic starts to set in. I'm definitely noticing a difference in the level it goes to and my ability to calm myself down. My family has noticed a huge difference in my behavior so far. I can't say enough! The support staff at Discover Health is amazing. I don't think you'll come across a friendlier group of people. I will continue to recommend Discover Health Functional Medicine Center to everyone I see, and I am so glad I have this resource in my life!

~ Nikki Wrobleski

CHAPTER FIVE

Hidden Infections and Toxins— the Foreign Invaders in Our Bodies

A world is not an ideology nor a scientific institution,
nor is it even a system of ideologies;
rather, it is a structure of unconscious relations
and symbiotic processes.
~ William Irwin Thompson

WE CAN'T LIVE WITH THEM, AND WE CAN'T LIVE WITHOUT THEM

At this point, it should be clear that the purpose of your immune system is to protect you from any foreign or dangerous entity that enters your body. It is your defense system and has many layers or branches to it. It should also be understood that when your immune system is faced with an overabundance of irritations or invaders, it is going to become hyperreactive and hypersensitive. An overreactive immune system leads a person down the path toward chronic inflammation and autoimmunity.

Remember, three things need to be present for anyone to develop an autoimmune disease in which their immune system turns against their own tissues and sees the tissue as foreign:

1. Genetic susceptibility
2. Barrier dysfunction, such as leaky gut
3. Environmental triggers

We do not have any control over the genetic susceptibility we are born into, but we are in control of our daily choices and the environment we create for ourselves. In Chapter Two, some of the most common environmental factors in our lives that are modifiable were presented:

- Food sensitivities or allergies
- Stress
- Relationships
- Allergens other than foods
- Recreational drugs
- Infections
- Toxins

In Chapter Three, we expanded on how food allergies or sensitivities can be an environmental trigger that irritates your immune system and leads down the path toward chronic inflammation and autoimmunity. We also explained how doing a comprehensive elimination diet for three weeks is the way to empower yourself to identify your individual food sensitivities.

In Chapter Four, we explored how stress can be an important environmental trigger for hyperreactivity and hypersensitivity of your immune system. We also explored how your perception and emotional response to the challenges in your life are what truly increase your stress. We provided some daily exercises to empower you to work on changing your perception toward more gratitude, compassion, and thankfulness.

In this chapter, let's continue to explore other categories of environmental triggers that disrupt the balance of your defenses.

We Live in a Symbiotic Relationship With Bugs

Back in Chapter Two, we introduced the concept that your microbiome is very connected to your overall health and the function of your immune system. We have a symbiotic relationship with bacteria: we all have two to three pounds of bacteria living in our colon at any given time, and we need them to survive. A good example of this symbiotic relationship between us and our microbiome occurs whenever we eat fiber.

Fiber is found in any plant-based food such as fruits, vegetables, and grains. The human digestive tract is not equipped to digest fiber, but the beneficial bacteria that live in our colon can digest fiber. They digest fiber for us, and when they do, they produce something we need called *short-chain fatty acids*. These short-chain fatty acids are what the cells that line our intestines use as fuel. So, this is what we mean by "we can't live without them."

But, as was explained in Chapter Two, you need to feed your gut microbiome healthy foods in order to promote a beneficial environment for a neighborhood full of health-producing bacteria rather than infectious bacteria. This is also why we should not be so afraid to play in the dirt.

Over the last twenty years, we have become far too extreme in our antibacterial attitude. We have been taught to use too many antibacterial products: antibacterial soap, hand wipes, sanitizers, and developed a fear that any and all bacteria are dangerous to our health. This attitude has been the root cause for most of the autoimmune diseases in our world today.

Some Don't Belong

What about the bacteria or other organisms that do cause infection and disease?

Everyone has experienced some form of an acute infection in their lives. An acute urinary tract infection, bronchitis, or pneumonia, or infection of a cut in your skin are all examples of acute infections. These types of acute infections are typically caused by bacteria, but the common cold is caused by a virus. In addition to infectious bacteria, other invaders can attack your body. Viruses and mold or fungi are other microorganisms that can make us ill once they breach our barriers. It is these invasive, infectious microorganisms that are dangerous and the primary enemy that our immune system is supposed to attack and eradicate for us.

Sometimes, antibiotics are necessary when an acute infection is caused by bacteria that our immune system is not able to eradicate on its own. Acute infections typically make us ill suddenly, and when the immune system eradicates the infection, all the invading organisms are destroyed.

But, chronic infections can occur, and this means that invasive and infectious microorganisms are living in us over long periods of time. They invade and set up house in the neighborhoods of our microbiome. For example, gingivitis is chronic inflammation of the gums around your teeth. It is caused by an accumulation of bacterial plaque on teeth that leads to tooth decay. A dental plaque is an example of a biofilm. A biofilm is a collection of one or more types of microorganisms that can grow collectively on many different surfaces. In any wet environment, the microorganisms attach themselves to a surface and produce a sticky, gooey substance that connects them and protects them from outsiders.

We all know that dental plaques are bad for our teeth, and this is why we brush our teeth every day, use dental floss, and go the dental hygienist typically twice a year to scrape dental plaques away so that we do not develop gingivitis and tooth decay. But, what you may not know is that chronic gingivitis can be the root cause of other chronic systemic illnesses, such as heart disease, diabetes, and lung disease. This is because your immune system is constantly reacting to the invasive organisms living in the dental plaques, but it cannot fully penetrate the protective community they have created. This leads to constant activity by your immune system and inflammation that spreads to other parts of your body.

Promote the Good; Get Rid of the Bad

One of the best examples of a biofilm is pond scum. We have all seen what happens on top of stagnant water. A thick, smelly, and gooey film develops. This is a community of bacteria, fungi, and algae that live together for mutual benefit in a neighborhood. Now, not all biofilms are bad. It depends on whether the neighborhood is full of beneficial and health-promoting organisms or if it is full of infectious and dangerous organisms.

This is what I mean when I say: *You want the right gangs running your neighborhoods*. We want to eat a diet that not only is going to provide us with the right vitamins, minerals, and phytonutrients; but, also promote the right organisms to be populating and running our biofilms and our microbiome. This is why probiotic or fermented foods are so healthy. Kombucha, for example, is a probiotic sweet tea. It is not difficult to make, but in order to make it, you will need a *scoby*, which is an acronym for Symbiotic Culture Of Bacteria and Yeast. It is also synonymous with what is called *the mother* in the probiotic and fermented foods world. Probiotic foods provide us with biofilms that are filled with beneficial and health-promoting microorganisms for our microbiome.

Chronic Inflammatory Response Syndrome

Chronic Inflammatory Response Syndrome, or CIRS, is another example of how chronic infections can cause a person's immune system to be out of control. It occurs when the immune system is constantly needing to respond to too many biotoxins or neurotoxins that are produced in the body by mold or other microorganisms. People who are suffering from CIRS typically have a genetic weakness in detoxifying or excreting the toxins given off by these microorganisms.

It is estimated that 24 percent of the population has this genetic weakness.[6]

Symptoms of CIRS may include:

- Fatigue
- Pain
- Sleep disturbance
- Asthma or other breathing disorders
- Abdominal pain and bowel problems
- Impaired memory
- Emotional imbalance with mood swings and anxiety

---

6   theashbulletin.blogspotcom/2017/04/mold-illness.html.
  Hamilton, K. "Chronic Inflammatory Response Syndrome: What is It? Why Should We Care? What Does It Have to Do with Our Brain Function?" theashbulletin.blogspot.com. January 7, 2017. stayinghealthytoday.com/cirs-mold-brain-function-jill-carnahan-md

The typical routes of exposure for microorganisms that can cause CIRS are inhalation of molds in a water-damaged building, tick or spider bites, direct contact with contaminated water, or ingestion of reef fish contaminated with certain types of algae. As you can see, the underlying root cause of someone's chronic inflammation or autoimmunity could be due to a chronic infection that can cause a complex array of symptoms that linger for years and progress to more and more debilitating illness.

With all this being said about microorganisms, you can understand what is meant by the statement "We can't live with them and we can't live without them." And, there are so many aspects of our lifestyle or daily choices that will either promote strong and healthy biofilms or inflammation and autoimmune-producing biofilms in us.

KEEP YOUR DEFENSES STRONG
AND BALANCED

So, how do you keep your immune system functioning optimally?

First, you must have a positive and supportive relationship with your immune system, so it is knowledgeable enough about who belongs and who doesn't belong, who the good guys are and who the bad guys are. Then, when the bad guys show up, your defenses are in a better position to get rid of them. That's what it's all about: support and balance.

Exhausted Soldiers Make Mistakes

If your immune system is always faced with invaders — such as bacteria, viruses, mold, or yeast — as well as a collection of other negative environmental irritants, your police force and soldiers are going to be exhausted, and they are going to make mistakes.

If you do not keep your defenses strong and well trained, then the invasive microorganisms are going to infiltrate the systems of your body. Let me explain another example of how smart some of the microorganisms can be. There's a process called *molecular mimicry*. Molecular mimicry is when the pathogens or microorganisms that enter your body evolve their protein structure to look similar to the protein structure of some of the cells and the organs in your own body. They can change their structure to look like a nerve cell, a muscle cell, or like a thyroid cell.

Your immune system's job is to find the imposters.

"Wait a minute," your police and soldiers say when they see the invaders, "that doesn't look normal. That's not right. That doesn't belong here."

Then what do they do?

They attack.

They attack the invading cells, but there's a problem. Let's say the invaders are attached to your thyroid gland. Because of the molecular mimicry, they look like all the other thyroid cells.

Your immune system does its job and attacks the invaders, but it also attacks healthy thyroid cells, which initiates the autoimmune process. Your immune system attacks and destroys your own thyroid gland.

In the journal *Nature,* authors C. Erec Stebbins and Jorge E. Galan write, "Microbial organisms have evolved a mechanism of concealment, similar to that of higher organisms such as the African praying mantis, or the chameleon, who camouflage themselves so they can mimic their background as not to be recognized by others."[7]

Do you see that microorganisms are very smart?

They are going to hide and camouflage themselves within your body. If you are not promoting an optimal and healthy immune system, then you're not supporting your air force, you're not supporting your

7   Stebbens, C. E. and J. E. Galan. "Structural Mimicry in Molecular Virulence." *Nature* (16 August 2001). 412; 701–705. DOI: 10.1038/35089000

police, you're not communicating and giving them the right information. The invaders will hide better; your soldiers are going to be exhausted, and they're going to make more mistakes. You're going to have more chronic disease and more autoimmune disease.

A Strong Immune System Is Better Able to Identify Insiders from Outsiders: Even the Hidden Can Be Found

In order to keep your immune system functioning optimally, there must be good communication throughout the different systems or communities of cells throughout your body. An immune system that develops in too clean or sterile an environment may be less educated and more prone to errors in discrimination.

To stay as healthy as possible doesn't mean you need to distance yourself from bacteria and pathogens completely; don't use antibacterial products all the time or fear coming into contact with germs. You want to play in the dirt! It's healthy to play in the dirt and be exposed to good bugs, also at times *bad* bugs, so that your immune system can learn. Your immune system needs to be in good communication with your whole body. You need to educate your immune system, and your immune system needs to educate you. It's important for a good community relationship.

I had an experience once that I think is a good analogy of different community relationships and how they can promote separation and miscommunication or openness and positive communication. I live in a small tourism community in the mountains of New Hampshire. One day, my two children and I went to a Kindness Day, when an author who wrote a book about kindness visited our community.

When we got there, we were told, "Alright, for the next four hours, we want you to go out and do random acts of kindness in the community."

I asked my kids, "What do you guys want to do?"

They said, "We want to go home and make some cookies, and we want to bring them to the firefighters in the fire department, and we want to bring some to the police department, and say, 'Thank you for all that you do.' "

So, we did that. We went home and we made cookies.

We went to the fire department first. When we arrived, the garage door was open, and there were a few people around cleaning the fire trucks and working in the garage.

We walked right in, we brought our cookies and some balloons, and we said, "We want to give this to you folks because you do such wonderful things in our community and protect us, and we just want to say thank you."

They all came right over, they gave us hugs, and it was great. It was really neat, and we left feeling joyful and more connected to the firefighters in our community. Then we got back in our car, and we went to the police department.

When we arrived at the police department, we couldn't quite figure out how to get in. It looked like a fort. It looked like an armory. When we finally figured out how to get in the door, we walked into a five-by-five–foot space. There were three doors. The walls were cement, the doors were metal, and we weren't sure if we should be in there or if we'd ever get out again. There was one window that was very thick and darkly colored, so we weren't sure what to do.

Then we realized there was a button on the wall. We pushed the button on the wall, and then a few moments later, this voice asked, "Can I help you?"

We said, "We're here to give to whoever's on duty some cookies and balloons to say thank you for what you do, as today is kindness day here in the valley."

"Alright. Don't know if anybody's in the office but hold on."

The voice went away. We stood there in silence for quite some time, feeling more and more uncomfortable and wondering whether we should leave or stay. A few minutes later, a doorknob started to turn on one of the doors. A gentleman stepped out. He was in his police uniform. He stood there sternly.

We said, "We'd like to give you these cookies and these balloons to say thank you for what you do."

He kind of looked at us, as if we were strange, then he said, "Alright."

At this point, I was intrigued by the difference between our experience at the fire department and here at the police department, so I decided to continue to play with this interaction. I smiled to myself and said, "Can we also give you a hug to say thanks for what you do?"

The police officer started to look all around and then looked back at us and said, "Is this like a Candid Camera thing or something?"

I use this story as an analogy. In many of our communities today the police are more separate and removed from our neighborhoods. The days of police officers walking daily through our towns and interacting closely with everyone who lives in the different neighborhoods has changed. An *us versus them* mentality seems to be prevalent today between many citizens and the police force within their community. This makes it much more difficult for the police to do their jobs because if they are not in good communication or interaction with the community, it makes it hard to recognize who is dangerous and who is safe.

If they are not out and about in the neighborhoods, then they are not going to notice or be aware of who belongs and who doesn't. They are not going to develop an educated level of tolerance within the melting pot of our communities, and this leads to hypervigilance and hyperreactivity, similar to an immune system that is hypervigilant and hyperreactive. Mistakes are bound to occur.

CHOICES THAT STRENGTHEN OR WEAKEN DEFENSES

The final category of environmental triggers that can disrupt your immune system and initiate the imbalances that lead to chronic inflammation and autoimmunity are toxins. We are all exposed to toxins. Some we consciously choose to expose ourselves to such as cigarettes, alcohol, or other recreational drugs; but, many we are not as aware of, such as industrialized chemicals, pollutants, and pesticides. There are more than 7 million recognized chemicals in existence, and approximately 80,000 are in common use. And even more concerning is the fact that tests on blood from the umbilical cord of newborn babies found 287 chemicals that consisted of pesticides, consumer product ingredients, and wastes from burning coal, gasoline, and garbage. Of the 287 chemicals found, 180 of them are known to cause cancer in humans or animals.[8]

Food Is Information

Most of the food we buy today is highly processed and full of additives and chemicals. For example, the food in boxes on the shelves of our grocery stores is full of trans-fats and hydrogenated fats, which are artificial fats that are inexpensive to create and increase the shelf life of the foods. Now it is well known that these fats can be a root cause to the underlying chronic inflammation that causes heart disease.

Industrialized farming or agribusiness, like all big business, has a primary goal of mass production and big profits. In this industry, the growth of fruits and vegetables involves fertilizers, pesticides, and genetically modifying seeds to produce bigger yields. The industrialized raising of animals or fish for consumption involves growth hormones, antibiotics,

8   "Body Burden: The Pollution in Newborns." Environmental Working Group. July 14, 2005. ewg.org/research/body-burden-pollution-newborns#.W00DVi2ZM6g

and extremely inhumane living conditions and slaughtering practices.

If you are eating a diet high in packaged and processed foods and industrialized meats or fish, then you are feeding yourself and your family food that is deficient in vitamins, minerals, and phytonutrients; but also full of dangerous chemicals that are possibly the root cause of your chronic inflammation and autoimmunity.

In order to empower yourself and provide your body and your immune system with more healthy food, you could start to make some of the following choices:

- Purchase real food from the periphery of the grocery store: fruits, vegetables, meat, eggs, and so on.

- Learn about the *Clean Fifteen* and the *Dirty Dozen*: fruits and vegetables grown with the least versus the most pesticides so that you know which ones you need to buy organic and which you may not have to.

- Buy foods labeled non-Genetically Modified (non-GMO) or Organic. Only plants grown from organic seeds are truly non-GMO.

- Buy grass-fed meats or wild-caught fish.

Endocrine Disruptors in Your Environment

Another category of toxic chemicals in the food industry or other commercial products are *endocrine disruptors*. These interfere with your endocrine system, which is the system of your body that deals with all your hormones. This includes your thyroid and adrenal glands, pancreas, ovaries, testicles, and pituitary gland. When endocrine disruptors are ingested, absorbed, or inhaled, they interfere with the production, action, and elimination of your hormones. They can raise or deplete levels of estrogen and testosterone, which when out of balance, can initiate inflammation or immune imbalance and create big problems for your health.

Here are some examples of sources of endocrine disruptors that are in your daily environment:

- Bisphenol A, also known as BPA, found in the lining of metal cans for food storage

- Plasticides, found in food wraps

- Phthalates, found in skin lotions and nail polish

- Parabens, found in cosmetics, makeup, body creams, and lotions

- Triclosan, found in antibacterial soaps

All these toxins are in our everyday world, but you can become educated on how to avoid them by making more informed consumer choices. At the end of this chapter, I will educate you about the Environmental Working Group, which is a nonprofit organization that can help.

Heavy Metals

The most common heavy metals that can be the root cause for chronic inflammation and disease include mercury, lead, arsenic, and cadmium. Iron, magnesium, potassium, zinc, and selenium are minerals from our environment that we all need to be healthy; but the heavy metals are disruptive to our health.

You may be exposed to heavy metals more than you realize. All fish, for example, even though very healthy for you, contain mercury and therefore should not be eaten more than twice per week on a regular basis. The level of mercury in any fish also depends on the size of the fish and how much it eats smaller fish that add to its mercury load. Shark and swordfish, for example, would have much higher loads of mercury than sardines or salmon.

Another method of exposure to heavy metals is in your water supply. For example, I have had a number of patients who were not optimally improving their health, no matter how many lifestyle improvements they made. We tested them for heavy metals and found high levels of arsenic. New Hampshire is called the Granite State and granite naturally contains arsenic. Once these patients realized this and installed a filter for their water system, their health began to improve.

Common sources for heavy metals include:

- Fertilizers
- Water supply
- Industrial waste and car emissions
- Foods
- Toys (color enhancers or anticorrosive agents used on them)
- Paints

Environmental Working Group

The *Environmental Working Group* is a nonprofit, nonpartisan organization dedicated to protecting human health and the environment. Their mission is to empower people to live healthier lives in a healthier environment. They have a wonderful website, EWG. org, that is an excellent resource for learning how to improve your health and avoid environmental triggers. For example, you can learn about the *Dirty Dozen* and the *Clean Fifteen,* mentioned earlier in this chapter. The Dirty Dozen is a list of the top twelve foods that are the most pesticide-laden foods in the farming industry. You do not want to purchase these fruits or vegetables conventionally grown; you need to buy them organically grown. The Clean Fifteen are the fifteen fruits and vegetables that are the least pesticide-laden; therefore, you can buy these conventionally grown and save some money.

Other features of EWG.org include the shopper's guides to cosmetics, cleaners, and foods. Once on the page of the website for one of these guides, simply enter the name of a specific product into their search field and the product will be rated as green: meaning go ahead and buy it, it is healthy for you and free of toxins; yellow: meaning you may want to think about buying it; and red: meaning it is highly toxic and you should leave it on the shelf and run away from it.

You Have the Power

In this chapter, the focus has been on how chronic infections from pathogenic microorganisms and toxins — such as pesticides, fertilizers, endocrine disruptors, and heavy metals — can disrupt your immune system and cause it to become hypersensitive, hyperreactive and hypervigilant. In our world today, many environmental triggers are destroying the protective barriers in our bodies and initiating an immune response; but this immune response is never-ending and chronic to the point that many of our immune systems are out of control, making mistakes and attacking the self.

This is a grim situation for many people, but there is hope because you have the power to shift your daily environment and empower yourself. You have the power to educate yourself. You have the power to make choices to eat foods that feed a healthy microbiome and therefore decrease or eliminate the infectious microorganisms. You have the power to avoid toxins and to detoxify your body and your environment. You have the power to make the choices to avoid the bad and promote the good so that your immune system is strong, not exhausted, communicating properly, and balanced enough to restore and optimize your health.

I came to Discover Health because I have Lyme disease. I learned about Trish Murray, DO, and Functional Medicine and I thought I'd give it a try. I felt so much better! I started feeling less joint pain, I started feeling more energy, I started feeling less brain fog. Having something like Lyme disease and going into a new program, there were really specific things that made me say, "Wow, I don't feel [discomfort] anymore!" and it's because of what I am doing here at Discover Health Functional Medicine Center, Inc.

~ Annie Pravanzano

Conclusion

Chronic inflammation and hypervigilance of the immune system in response to numerous environmental irritants is the main reason why society is faced with the chronic disease epidemic of our time. The function of the immune system is to defend and protect you from outside invaders. It is your military or police force, and it is complex and has multiple layers. When the soldiers of the immune system run out of control and an autoimmune disease is diagnosed there are three main reasons for it:

1. Genetic Susceptibility
2. Barrier Dysfunction or a breakdown in the fort
3. Environmental trigger(s)

This book's focus is to educate and empower you on the root causes of chronic inflammation and autoimmunity. The possible barrier dysfunctions and environmental triggers are explored, and steps are offered that you can implement to modify your lifestyle to heal your fort, quiet your triggers, and balance your defenses.

The first step back to health is to identify which environmental irritants you think are your biggest triggers and start to make some of the changes suggested to modify your daily environment.

The different categories of environmental triggers include:

- Food Sensitivities or Allergens
- Stress
- Infections
- Toxins

Most people will have a combination of imbalances leading from a number of these categories. Ask yourself numerous questions:

- *Are the foods I'm eating proinflammatory?*

- *How do I perceive the challenges in my life, and how am I managing my stress?*

- *Am I getting enough rest?*

- *Do I have a practice daily to quiet my mind?*

- *Do I exercise regularly?*

- *Am I aware of the chemicals in my daily life from my food, cosmetics, cleaners?*

- *Am I taking any action to detoxify my body or my mind?*

- *Am I constantly taking another pill to try and quiet another symptom?*

- *Do I work or live in a water-damaged building?*

- *Do I have gingivitis or any other chronic infection?*

Once you have identified for yourself the area of your life that you think needs to be worked on and improved the most, then review some of the suggestions given in this book and step on the road to restoring your health. Start with one goal at a time, make an action plan, and carry it out. Talk with your family and your friends about your goal and your plan and ask if they would like to join you on this journey or at least support you in this process.

If you are unsure how to get started or you are feeling overwhelmed, we can help. You can reach out to me and my staff at Discover Health Functional Medicine Center. My website is discoverhealthfmc.com, and you can schedule a free thirty-minute consult with one of us directly on the website if you wish to discuss our services and how we can help.

Also on my website are numerous other avenues for more education to empower you:

- Health Library: full of free educational materials including blogs, podcasts, exercise videos.

- A free internet course entitled "10 Ways in 10 Days to Stop Your Suffering and Live a Pain-Free Life"

- A free talk providing an overview of our most intensive and supportive service program, the D.E.N.T.™ Program, to help you put a dent in your chronic disease.

- Discover Health Practice Membership: this membership gives you access to all the empowering educational materials I've ever created.

- In the shop, numerous individual online courses are available, such as The Detox Plus Program discussed in Chapter Three.

Next Steps

1. Realize that Your Life Depends on You! There is HOPE! And with the right education, coaching, mentoring, and support, you can restore and optimize your health.

2. Select one aspect of your lifestyle you are going to work on improving, then go back to the chapter in this book that discusses actions to take and start implementing them. Make a plan and stick to it.

3. Go to my website, discoverhealthfmc.com, and keep learning, or schedule your free thirty-minute consult.

4. Go to my Facebook page "Discover Health Functional Medicine Center" and join our Facebook Group. It is a place where you can interact with like-minded people trying to improve their health and their lives just like you. There, you can get your most burning questions answered.

About the Author

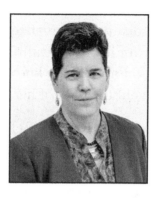

Patricia (Trish) Murray, DO, is a highly accomplished physician who has been certified in four different medical specialties, including internal medicine, osteopathic manipulative medicine, energy medicine, and functional medicine. All of this after teaching for a decade in public education and, at the age of thirty-eight years old, completing medical school in the top 10 percent of her graduating class.

Dr. Murray has designed numerous courses in Osteopathic Manipulative Medicine and has taught hundreds of physicians in continuing education programs for more than ten years. Her live, as well as internet-based, nationally accredited courses are sought after by physicians internationally.

As the result of a personal injury that traditional medical therapies could not help when she was a young athlete, as well as experiencing the anguish of losing her mom to Alzheimer's disease long before her mother's physical death, Trish realized that she had to take responsibility for her own health. Her mission has been to seek and accumulate the knowledge necessary to heal and to prevent the path of her genetics.

Trish is the founder of Discover Health Functional Medicine Center and has had the honor of instructing and supporting thousands of patients through their personal journey to restore and optimize their health from a multitude of chronic diseases.

Trish lives in the White Mountains of New Hampshire with her partner, Elaine, who is a forest ranger. She can walk out her back door and hike to her heart's content. Her stepdaughter, Shea, who has always been the artist in the family, has blossomed into an amazing hair stylist. Stepson Ben is in college studying environmental science and conservationism. Trish's most joyful moments have come from spending quality time helping nurture these two amazing people and watching them flourish. She is looking forward to being a grandma someday, whenever they choose to have children.

35659581R00076